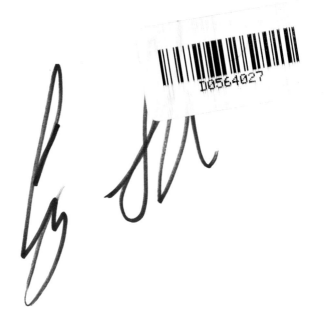

The DEFINITIVE GUIDE TO YOUTH ATHLETIC
STRENGTH, CONDITIONING & PERFORMANCE

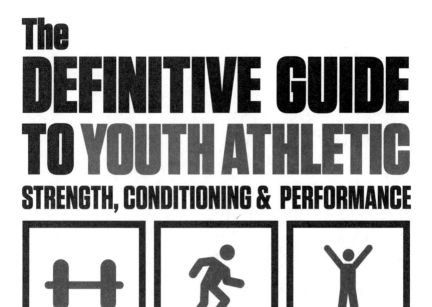

Published by CelebrityPress™, Orlando, FL
A division of The Celebrity Branding Agency®

Celebrity Branding® is a registered trademark
Printed in the United States of America.

ISBN: 9780983947042
LCCN: 2011945053

This publication is designed to provide accurate and authoritative information with regard to the subject matter covered. It is sold with the understanding that the publisher is not engaged in rendering legal, accounting, or other professional advice. If legal advice or other expert assistance is required, the services of a competent professional should be sought. The opinions expressed by the authors in this book are not endorsed by CelebrityPress™ and are the sole responsibility of the author rendering the opinion.

Most CelebrityPress™ titles are available at special quantity discounts for bulk purchases for sales promotions, premiums, fundraising, and educational use. Special versions or book excerpts can also be created to fit specific needs.

For more information, please write:

CelebrityPress™,

520 N. Orlando Ave, #2
Winter Park, FL 32789
or call 1.877.261.4930

Visit us online at www.CelebrityPressPublishing.com

The
DEFINITIVE GUIDE
TO YOUTH ATHLETIC
STRENGTH, CONDITIONING & PERFORMANCE

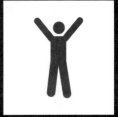

Contents

CHAPTER 1

Mistakes Coaches Make With Young Athletes

By Pat Rigsby & Nick Berry

Serving young athletes is one of the most powerful things that any adult can do. As a coach, not only can you have a profound impact on the child's success in their respective athletic endeavors, but more importantly, you can make an indelible impact on the children you are coaching – in all aspects of their lives.

However, along with this wonderful opportunity to empower young people, there also comes significant responsibility. There is a responsibility to not only deliver quality technical advice and guidance, but also to treat young athletes with a respect and attitude, which helps to instill a lifelong passion for physical activity.

With that in mind, here are a few common mistakes coaches made when working with young athletes, and some insight as to how you can correct or avoid them.

MISTAKE #1 - USING EXERCISE AS A PUNISHMENT

Young people play sports and are active because it's fun. Our role as coaches and mentors is to set them up for as much fun as possible in the hopes that they continue playing from year to year. Young athletes eventually become adults, and the experiences they have as kids will play a major role in whether or not they choose to be active or not later in life, and how they treat the young people in their lives.

Thinking that physical exercise is punishment will create a negative attitude toward it, and will lead the young athlete to try to avoid that exercise.

A better approach is to always tie exercise to the benefits that it yields, from the immediate gratification of the fun associated with the activity, to the athletic or physical benefits that the exercise will yield over time. Remember – your job as a coach isn't to get your athletes tired, anyone can do that. *Your job is to help them become better.*

MISTAKE #2 – TREATING YOUNG ATHLETES LIKE MINIATURE ADULTS

It doesn't matter how big, strong, or coordinated a young athlete is, he or she is not an adult. Young athletes are still maturing mentally, physically and socially. They're still growing and developing. Because of this, they require a specific approach to both programming and style of coaching. What's appropriate for a young athlete should be determined by their movement mechanics and their level of physical development as well as their psychosocial maturity, and it is never the same as what's appropriate for an adult.

A more sound approach to programming and coaching young people is to study performance training and coaching education that is specifically developed for young people – like that offered through the International Youth Conditioning Association. The educational information and resources provided through the IYCA is specific to young athletes and the coaches that serve them. You can learn more at: www.IYCA.org.

MISTAKE #3 – SPORT SPECIALIZATION FOR YOUNG ATHLETES

One of the most common mistakes made with young athletes in our society currently is the specialization of a sport at a young age. Adults mistakenly think that early specialization will lead to long-term success for a particular sport, while the reality is that the opposite is often true. Specialization has been shown to increase the risk of injury and burnout in young athletes, while participating in a variety of sports and physical activities has seemed to decrease the occurrence of both of these problems. Young athletes should be exposed to a variety of sports and exercise activities in a variety of settings with different young people – so that they can discover what they enjoy while maximizing their physical, psychological, and social development.

MISTAKE #4 – FOCUSING ON THE WRONG THINGS

All too often adults try to impose adult-type objectives on young people instead of allowing them to focus on the things that young athletes should be focused on. Whether it be having a young athlete focus on technique when they could be developing power or focusing on drills instead of developing skills, adults should allow kids to have their own objectives for the sports and activities that they are involved in. Not only will this improve their experience in the moment, but it will improve their long-term development as well.

MISTAKE #5 – 'WINNING' ABOVE ALL ELSE

There is nothing more pathetic than adults trying to live vicariously through their young children, determined to win 'Championships' with 9 year olds, dragging their children around the country with U8 travel teams, and gloating about winning at a stage when sports should be about activity, learning and fun.

This approach has led to a higher than ever before attrition rate within youth sports, and in turn, has been a significant factor in the growing youth obesity rates and decreased activity levels within the youth population.

As a coach of young athletes, your job is to help young people get better. To teach them and instill in them a lifelong passion for sport and physical activity. Not to weed out kids because they weren't 'early developers' or didn't show proficiency for a particular sport at an early age. If you provide an experience that causes a young athlete to be excited about participating the next year, you've won.

MISTAKE #6 – NOT BEING POSITIVE

Along the same lines with mistakes numbers 4 and 5, all too often coaches and parents focus on the negative with young athletes rather than 'catching them doing something right.' Good coaches give young athletes a chance to succeed and help them understand what is expected of them. In turn, they may be more likely to see mistakes as part of the learning process and use those mistakes as a means of enhancing their personal motivation. Remember, the real motivators for young athletes are to have fun, gain social acceptance and to develop and demonstrate competence – in that order. If you remove the 'fun' and degrade them with regular negative enforcement, you will lose their interest.

MISTAKE #7 – NOT LEARNING ABOUT KIDS

Yes, coaches can learn as much from kids as kids can learn from them. Study kids and you'll find that coaches aren't what / who motivates them. It's the game, the challenge, the competition and their peers.

As a coach, you're getting to witness first-hand human growth and development. These young athletes are developing their own self-concept – developing socially, mentally and physically. By learning about the critical learning periods young people go through and how you can best support the children you coach, you'll be much more successful in helping them improve and enjoy their experience.

Being a coach with good intentions and a willingness to work with young people is not enough. The education of coaches is the foundation of long-term athlete development. Coaches need to not only learn from their own experiences, but also study the information that is available about long-term youth athlete development. The most successful youth coaches are willing to change old habits and be taught new skills. By learning more about the art and science of coaching young people, coaches will be better prepared to help their athletes become the best they can be – by adapting to what is best for the children they serve.

Sport and physical activity are such wonderful things that should be part of every young person's life. They teach values. They teach competition. They improve health, self-confidence and so much more. And above all else, they're fun. My suggestion to you is to allowing the focus to go back to the kids and what's best for them. They don't need to be great to participate. They don't need to win championships and become the next Major League All-Star. They certainly don't need to give parents and coaches something to brag about or carry the burden of our own hopes and dreams. All they have to do is enjoy.

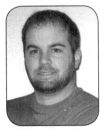

About Nick

Nick Berry has spent his entire career as an Entrepreneur in the Fitness industry. His experience has given him the opportunity to become a Business Coach and Consultant, and co-owner of dozens of other businesses – which have allowed him to help thousands of other small business owners, both in and out of the Fitness industry.

Nick co-founded, co-owns, and continues to build the Athletic Revolution™ and Fitness Revolution™ franchise systems. Athletic Revolution™ (www.myathleticrevolution.com) is a youth-based sports performance franchise which began in 2009 and currently has over 30 franchise units. Fitness Revolution™ (www.fitnessrevolutionfranchise.com) is an adult fitness franchise, which began in January 2011, and currently has over 50 franchise units.

Nick partnered with Pat Rigsby in 2005 and they continue to operate Fitness Consulting Group, (www.fitbusinessinsider.com) from which they offer their Fitness business consulting programs. He has helped build and co-owns the International Youth Conditioning Association, which is considered the premier international authority on youth conditioning and athletic development (www.iyca.org). He also was a co-author of the International Best Selling *Total Body Breakthroughs* book in the spring of 2011.

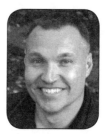

About Pat

Pat Rigsby is an author, consultant and fitness entrepreneur as well as the Co-Owner of over a dozen businesses within the fitness industry. He and Nick Berry's company, the Fitness Consulting Group, is the leading business development organization in the Fitness industry. The Fitness Consulting Group provides resources, coaching programs and consulting, to give you everything you need to start or grow your personal training or fitness-related business.

In addition to his business coaching and consulting work, Pat is also the Co-Owner of two of the fastest growing franchises in the fitness industry, Fitness Revolution and Athletic Revolution.

Fitness Revolution is the leading training-based franchise in the world and designed specifically to allow quality fitness professionals to develop great businesses. You can learn more at: www.fitnessrevolutionfranchise.com.

Athletic Revolution is the top youth fitness and sports performance franchise in the world today and the leading resource for long-term athletic development for kids ages 6-18. You can learn more about Athletic Revolution at: www.myathleticrevolution.com.

Pat also has helped build and co-owns the International Youth Conditioning Association, which is considered the premier international authority on youth conditioning and athletic development (www.iyca.org).

You can read Pat's popular newsletter serving over 65,000 fitness professionals worldwide, or learn more about all of his offerings at: www.fitbusinessinsider.com.

CHAPTER 2

Physical Fitness Section

By Kristy Lee Wilson

As a young child I would constantly flip myself around my parents house. I'd flip over the couch, off the walls, from the trampoline into the pool. Anything I could climb on, or flip myself over, I would. When I turned five, my mother decided she would take me to gymnastics classes to have someone teach me how to do this properly so that I wouldn't break something in her house. I was always hitting the coffee tables and other furniture that would get in my way around the house, but my mom wasn't worried about me … she was more worried about what I would break in her house.

As a five year old, I loved the sport of gymnastics. I couldn't get enough of it. I'd go to practice, go home and practice more. I'd stand on my head to watch TV. I'd even watch my parents play grass hockey and football standing on my head! I was always upside down and flipping around any chance I got.

By the time I was eight, I was winning most competitions I'd entered as well as having won a few state championship medals. One particular competition I won changed my life. I was competing at a local meet and the Australian Women's National Gymnastics Coach was there. I didn't know it at the time, but she had her eyes glued on me the entire meet. After the competition she spoke to my coach and asked if she could spend a few minutes with me and took me through a few 'tests.' I guess I passed because she invited me to a national camp with 64 other young promising gymnasts from all over the country. We spent a week at camp and she then selected just 4 girls back for a second week. I spent the second week with my coach and was then offered a 3-month scholarship to train at the Australian Institute of Sport with the best gymnasts in the country. What a dream come true for an eight year old! To be offered a scholarship to the AIS you had to be 12 years old, however the coach saw so much potential and talent in me she made an exception. I was over the moon and ready to go. My dream of representing Australia and competing in the Olympic Games was coming true.

Little did I know what the next eight years would entail, and that my dream would be shattered shortly before the 1996 Olympic Games – due to a knee injury requiring me to undergo three knee surgeries in the space of six months as a 14 year old.

After being offered and accepting my full time scholarship at the Australian Institute of Sport, I moved states as an eight year old to start training and preparing to achieve my goal of competing in the 1996 Olympic Games. As an eight year old, I would train eight hours a day, six days a week. Usually four hours in the morning and then another four to five hours at night. Between sessions I would go to school for a few hours.

Training was hard and there was a lot of frustration, yelling, and tears. This became a serious thing. No more having fun. I had to be serious. I was being weighed morning and night, yelled at if I wasn't the weight I was supposed to be, called fat, sent to the sauna, told I shouldn't eat. Beautiful gymnasts were skinny and looked like little girls.

Looking back, I don't know how I survived.

By the age of ten, I had developed what I soon would learn was known as an eating disorder. I became obsessed with food. I was petrified of food. I knew exactly how many sips of water would make the scale read 0.05kg heavier. I knew exactly how much most of the food I ate weighed. Sometimes I needed to eat, but then got so scared of what the scale would read so would then try to get rid of the food whether it be running or doing V-ups for hours, sleeping with 3 sweat suits on and my electric blanket on 40 degrees, purging multiple times in the space of an hour ... you name it, I tried it.

I don't remember the exact age, but at some point this all took a toll on me and I lost enjoyment for the sport. How could that happen? As a young child I couldn't get enough of the sport. Now as a teenager it felt like a chore. I was in constant pain, battling a severe eating disorder that would go on to haunt me for the next 15 years, and was constantly being yelled at, belittled and told I was too weak ... I'd never make it.

The sound of my alarm clock on the days I knew I had to go to the track to run 400 meter sprints would shoot terror through my veins. I would always pray for rain these days. Until a few years ago, that same sound would *still* have the same effect. If I heard an alarm on TV I would have to change the channel as quickly as possible. My days seemed to consist of being in fear, constant pain and exhaustion, battling my eating disorder and being frustrated that I could never doing anything right, even though I tried so hard.

What's interesting is that when I got injured and went through my knee surgeries, the thing I missed most was going to the gym to train. I really missed training and everything that went with it a lot, which is what made me get back in the gym and start training again. I had always loved training on trampoline as a gymnast so decided I would switch sports and see what else I could do. I tried my hand at trampoline, power tumbling and diving and quickly found my passion was still on the floor.

Competing in power tumbling was fun and a blessing in disguise because it led me to the Cirque du Soleil stage as a powertrack performer with Cirque's Orlando-based production 'La Nouba' for almost 10 years. Throughout this time, I went on to undergo three more surgeries, a severe back injury, and perhaps the worst part of my eating disorder. I fell into a dark hole and lost the desire to live for a while. Dealing with an eating disorder is really one of the toughest and ugliest things you can go through.

I am now fully recovered, healthy and taking my love for fitness and gymnastics to the fitness stage as a fitness competitor. Once you have gymnastics in your blood, you can really never get rid of it! So now here I am, teaching other young gymnasts how to be successful, prolong their gymnastic careers, and prevent the same struggles I went through.

From what I have learned from my own personal career as a gymnast and from training my own gymnasts, here are my top 5 ways to improve your performance and achieve success as a gymnast.

1. Condition Your Body Well

Pound-for-pound, gymnasts are some of the strongest athletes in the world. What gymnasts do with their bodies is beyond what's 'normal' for the human body. As a result, building a strong and balanced physique is essential for any gymnast. However, because weight and size does play a significant role in gymnastics, we want to train in a way where we can build strength and muscle without adding a lot of extra weight or bulk. The special strength needs of gymnasts mean that a strength-training program for gymnasts must be designed with the demands of the sport in mind.

I am constantly amazed by the conditioning, or lack of conditioning, programs given to the gymnasts I train. One eleven-year-old gymnast I've been working with for a while came to me one day with legs so sore she could barely walk. After asking her why she was so sore I learned her team was being made do the workout video *Insanity* before their skill practice. Yes, before their practice. Not only is *Insanity* totally irrelevant for gymnasts, but it is completely inappropriate for children!

The principle of specificity informs us that exercises used in practice should be similar to those exercises and movements that's are performed in routines. In addition, although the demands for gymnastics are similar for all gymnasts, the needs of each individual gymnast are different. Evaluating each individual gymnast is crucial so that valuable information can be obtained and a specific training program can be developed for the needs of each gymnast.

A well-rounded strength-training program for gymnasts will include working on muscular endurance, cardiovascular endurance, speed, agility, power, kinesthetic awareness, balance, and most importantly flexibility.

2. Stretch, Stretch, and Stretch!

Good flexibility is perhaps the biggest factor when it comes to achieving success as a gymnast. Gymnasts are required to move their bodies through extreme positions which would be extremely difficult, if not impossible, to do without adequate flexibility or range of motion in the major joints of the body.

While there are some structural and functional limitations that can affect flexibility, a good stretching program can help a gymnast achieve their flexibility potential and should include stretches for the major joint areas such as the ankle, knee, hip, back, shoulder, elbow and wrist. Of these, perhaps the most important joints requiring optimal flexibility (that need to be developed for the gymnast), include the hip, shoulder and back.

There are numerous stretching methods such as self–myofascial release, static stretching, and dynamic stretching that can be implemented to help a gymnast improve flexibility. However, like strength training, the best way to improve a gymnast's flexibility is to develop a stretching program specifically for the individual needs of each gymnast.

3. Practice Injury Prevention

The most common injuries in gymnastics include overuse injuries, strains, and sprains, and generally involve the achilles, ankle, wrist, elbow, back and shoulder. However, serious and traumatic injuries can occur as well. The good news is that many gymnastics injuries can be prevented with appropriate conditioning programs, learning correct technique and progressions, and also allowing enough rest for a previous injury to fully heal.

If an injury is suffered, trying to push through that injury, especially when it is in the acute phase, without giving it the time it needs to heal will most likely result in the injury becoming worse, perhaps leading to surgery or even a career-ending injury. Injuries definitely are frustrating and take away time from training. However, if you truly want a long career as a gymnast, when it comes to injuries you need to be smart with how you deal with them. The 'no pain, no gain' concept does not work in this case.

All gymnasts should perform a proper warm up and cool down prior to competition or training sessions. Injury prevention exercises can and should be incorporated into your training program each day. Exercises that are targeted to strengthen the ankles, wrist, core, and shoulder are great additions to an injury-prevention program for gymnasts.

4. Practice Proper Progressions

It has been documented that the number one cause of injuries in gymnastics is because the gymnast wasn't properly prepared or 'ready' to perform a certain skill. Progressions are essential to learning any skill, and following the proper progression sequences is vital. For example, a gymnast should not be taught a back handspring before they have mastered a handstand.

I constantly see coaches trying to get gymnasts to perform the more difficult skills before they have mastered the basics. Without a solid foundation, building the walls, then a roof, a house will fall down quickly. Make sure you can not only perform the basics, but can perform them consistently with correct technique, before you move on to learning a more advanced progression or skill. Many unnecessary injuries could be prevented by progressing skills more appropriately. Of course, it's nice to be able to do the harder skills, but at what cost to the athlete?

Gymnastics is a dangerous sport, so we need to be smart and make it as safe as possible. Don't push a gymnast who is not yet physically ready to perform certain skills. Focus on improving the basics, or current progression, and the final result will be worth the little extra time spent there.

5. Practice Good Sports Nutrition

Whether we want to admit it or not, eating disorders and disordered eating are a big part of gymnastics. In gymnastics, weight is a common topic heard around gyms and coaches commonly suggest to their gymnasts that a low weight is desired if success as a gymnast is to be achieved. As a result, many young gymnasts turn to unhealthy methods, like myself, to achieve a low weight. While it is true that reducing body mass will perhaps lower the risk of injuries and stress on the joints, reducing weight through unhealthy methods actually places the gymnast at much greater risk of injury and early burnout.

To perform at our best we need to fuel our body with adequate energy and nutrients that meet the demands of training and improving strength. The focus of gymnastics should be on the training and conditioning rather than keeping weight low. A strong gymnast will be a good gymnast. Being strong makes it easier to master more advanced skills, it reduces fear of learning these skills, and also reduces risk of injury. The best way to improve strength and conditioning is through a good training program, but most importantly by consuming enough calories and nutrients to support the program.

Unhealthy athletes don't stay competitive for very long, so it is extremely important to eat enough of the right foods, consisting mostly of whole grains, fruits and vegetables, lean protein sources, and good fats, if your goal is to stay competitive as a gymnast and have a long career.

ABOUT KRISTY

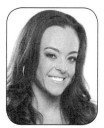

Kristy Lee Wilson is considered one of the premier experts on strength and conditioning for gymnasts. Kristy became an elite gymnast at the age of eight and for the past decade was wowing crowds nightly, performing with the world- renowned Cirque du Soleil as a power-track/trampoline artist in the Orlando - based production, "La Nouba."

Originally from Australia, Kristy made her mark in fitness at an extremely young age. At just eight years Kristy became the youngest athlete to ever be offered a scholarship to the Australian Institute of Sport. Kristy was one of Australia's top junior gymnasts, three-time Australian Power Tumbling Champion and Cirque du Soleil performer. When it comes to experience, there are very few fitness professionals who have the personal experience Kristy has. Kristy is also a sponsored athlete and fitness competitor.

As a fitness professional, Kristy Lee Wilson is highly respected and certified through the top strength and conditioning associations in the world – the National Academy of Sports Medicine, the National Strength and Conditioning Association, and the International Youth Conditioning Association. Kristy is also the founder and owner KLW Fitness. Kristy specializes in Sports Performance Enhancement - particularly in gymnastics, dance, cheerleading, and MMA, Corrective Exercise and Youth Fitness.

In 2011, Kristy won the Fitness America Universe Tour in Florida and was named Ms Fitness Florida. She was also recognized as a National Association of Professional Women's - Woman of the Year. Kristy is one of the Top 10 Fitness Expert's on Dr Oz's new health website Sharecare, and is an advisor for the Excellence Through Exercise Foundation. Kristy has been featured and published in publications such as USANA magazine, World Physique Magazine, Today & Tonight Magazine, and A Sky's the Limit Magazine, and is seen as a featured fitness expert on numerous health and fitness websites.

To learn more about Kristy Lee Wilson visit: www.kristywilson.com or contact: kristyleefitness@me.com.

CHAPTER 3

Understanding the Mind-Set of a Young Athlete

By Mike Pickles

During my professional experience as an strength and conditioning coach, I have learned one very important thing about an athlete's performance….. it's directly related to their mind-set regardless of how skilled they are. I realized this while working as an instructor at a summer recreation camp for youth ages 5-13 during my college years. The insight I gained motivated me to learn more from a human development course I took as part of my college program in Fitness and Health Promotion. What motivates youth and young athletes can sometimes be complex to understand, but I believe the answers lie within the environment where they grew up and how they were raised by their parents.

There is no doubt that what makes a special performance coach is the ability to relate to young athletes on their own level. Thinking back to our own childhood at different stages of our lives can help give us insight into what motivates the young athletes we coach. Think about how we viewed the world around us growing up, absorbing and analyzing information from every situational experience. These experiences, either good or bad, molded who we are today and, as a result, it's why we view ourselves the way we do. We're all products of our environment at every stage in life. Our beliefs change, our values change, we change how we feel about our confidence, self-esteem, and everything else involved in the evolution of our character.

Most adults often forget how they felt growing up, and sometimes expect kids to think the way they do. When kids act immaturely or misbehave we tend to ask the question, "What were you thinking?" or "Why did you do that?" The answer is they don't know, they're still learning, analyzing, trying to figure out who they are and where they fit in. Kids are kids, and it's important to understand that they're very vulnerable and often act in ways to attract attention for securing some kind of identity. Kids actually do have complex lives, where trying to manage school, friends, and everything else, is important for establishing their identity.

Understanding the mind-set of youth and young athletes is imperative to helping them believe in themselves, and provide the discipline that comforts their need to know they are cared about. I believe positive re-enforcement and constructive criticism will always be the most effective methods of support for young athletes to know that it's ok to make mistakes, because it makes them better. This has an enormous impact on the rest of their lives for developing character, not just as an athlete, but as a human being.

My education in human development has helped me reflect on my own life growing up as a young athlete. I remember my fears and insecurities prevented me from wanting to excel in sports although I was a great athlete. That vision of my past is what drives me today to empower my young athletes to believe in their potential for greatness.

My athletic background started at the early age of five, playing ice-hockey in a small town called Parry Sound, home of the great Bobby Orr. Ice-hockey was the dominant sport in my town where most parents hoped to see their kid in the NHL one day. I was a shy and quiet kid who was scared to be ridiculed or embarrassed, but had confidence in my ability to be good at what I did, and I scored goals. I remember always wanting to make plays by myself and didn't want anyone's help for some reason. I could figure out the game on my own, and despite the confidence I had in my abilities, I remember lacking the self-esteem.

My father was very supportive, and like most fathers, he wanted to see me get better and succeed. He gave me that little push to continue playing when my low self-esteem persuaded me not to. Why I lacked self-esteem I don't know, but I was always looking for a way out. One thing I remember was that I couldn't handle other kids making fun of me. My parents were never on the same page about empowering me to feel like nothing can get in my way of success. My mother said if I didn't want to keep playing ice-hockey then I didn't have to, and so I took the easy road out. They never forced anything upon me, but I think if they collectively gave me the reinforcement that I needed, I might have really excelled in hockey and built stronger self-esteem.

A few years later, my dad coached our soft-ball team, and for whatever reason, I didn't continue to play that for very long either. My father wanted to see me excel, but the lack of my mother's support comforted my insecurities. It's unfortunate for me that my parents didn't share the same views, because things could have been a lot different for my future as an athlete. What I remember most is how much I feared making mistakes, but it didn't stop me from playing many other sports growing up. I just loved having fun playing sports with my friends, but I needed someone to empower me to go all the way. I didn't even have a coach that inspired me enough to excel in one particular sport, so I didn't bother to do so. I was a highly-skilled athlete with low motivation to succeed, and that carried over into the rest of my life, where I felt that being just good enough at anything was ok.

When working with my young athletes, I constantly pay attention to how they act and respond to my coaching cues. I'm always more focused on the athletes who seem to be lost, goof around and act like they don't care to be a part of our training sessions. There are many reasons why young athletes have different mind-sets, and as performance coaches, we need to figure out why. It's our job to inspire the ones who don't care and guide the others who have the desire, but just lack the skills.

Adjusting my coaching style accordingly is the first thing I analyze, because if something doesn't work, I have to try a different approach to get my message across. As performance coaches, we can't expect every young athlete to respond the same way to our coaching cues and techniques. Regardless of how hard we try, some kids will never pay attention, and all we can do is our best. However, those athletes who show poor mind-set through lack of motivation are the ones we should pay more attention to..... for finding that connection and lifting up their spirit.

I've learned a great deal from the Head Coach of the football team I work with. I listen very carefully how he addresses the team and talks to them. He's very inspiring and has realistic expectations from his athletes based on their abilities. Working with most of the same kids for 6 years he knows them well, he knows each individual's mind-set and the team as a whole. He understands what these kids go through everyday growing up in school and at home. Adapting accordingly to the needs of his athletes, he shows great passion for the game and does his best to empower these kids. He knows that his message doesn't sink in for everyone, but that it's OK because some kids just aren't focused for many reasons.

Here's a story of a young athlete I've trained who had a mind-set for being determined to succeed at the challenges I presented to him. He had incredible drive and was very competitive in every nature, although he seemed very quiet and unsure about what to expect from our training sessions. I tested him by using different coaching techniques so I could get a better idea of what he expected from himself, if anything at all. By getting to know his parents better, I had a pretty good idea how to relate to him based on their influence. He was highly motivated, but just needed some guidance to improve his skill level by working on his mobility and flexibility first.

When I put him through a functional movement screen and had him perform basic athletic skills, I watched his frustration increase as he had a hard time performing certain components. Most kids don't like doing what they can't do, and that's understandable. This was a window of opportunity for me to reassure him that he was only going to get better, but it wasn't going to be easy. With every session he was learning how to overcome the adversity that challenged him, learning that patience and hard work pay off.

His flexibility and mobility improved during the first six weeks and helped him to perform a full deep squat. That gave him the confidence to jump completely over a 16 inch bench - which was exciting - considering in the first week he had trouble jumping onto a 6 inch platform. He became more excited about his training sessions because he could see his improvements. I gave him the task of designing his own training circuit in order to create a sense of ownership for his accomplishments, and it was gratifying to hear his mother mention how much he looked forward to training.

He had a good support system from his parents, but they also taught him that it takes hard work to become successful. I saw him completely change when his mom came to pick him up one day and we were on the last part of a circuit. He moved faster, decreasing his time and his technique at the power clean was perfect – generating more force than I ever saw before. He showed a great sense of pride for his accomplishments, and was excited that his mother just witnessed his progress. His confidence had become even stronger and that mind-set translated onto the playing field. I can only hope that the impact of my coaching will help him grow up believing in himself – to achieve anything in life and become a better person, not just a better athlete.

On the opposite end, and a much shorter story is that of an athlete I trained in the past who showed poor attitude and mind-set towards training. This athlete was lazy and complained about the hard work that was expected of her during our training sessions. She only cared about playing the game of her chosen sport, and just liked to boast that she had her own trainer. I got to learn that she had a hard time dealing with the adversities of competition and the pressure to succeed at the University level. When I got to know her parents better, I realized they were over-pampering and gave off a false sense of perfection where she could do no wrong.

Always making excuses and pointing the finger at someone else, this athlete carried a sense of entitlement. In realizing that, I demanded respect during training and set high expectations for her. I prescribed challenging exercises that I knew she wasn't good at so I could teach her how to deal with failure. I felt I'd be doing her no favours if I praised everything she did, and led her to believe she was perfect. On a positive note, we had many conversations where I shared my own experiences in life coping with ups and downs. I just hope she remembers those life lessons and can get through tough times when they happen, because life isn't perfect. This is one athlete that had a high potential to succeed or fail, depending on her mind-set.

In the end, I believe there can be many reasons for how an athlete's mind-set is developed, but think that parenting still plays a big role. Some talented athletes can still develop a strong mind-set and excel on their own terms – even in a negative and unsupportive environment. As well, some athlete's might display poor mind-set in sports even with very supportive parenting. What I've also seen before are those born into affluent families who never learn what hard work is all about, and end up failing in sports and in life, even if they're a good athlete.

"Success is a state of mind, knowing that you did the best you could possibly do, to be the best you are possibly capable of being."
~ John Wooden, UCLA Basketball Coach

THREE TIPS TO UNDERSTANDING THE MIND-SET OF A YOUNG ATHLETE.

1. Parents and team coaches cannot expect kids to conduct themselves as adults, simply because they are not, and remember adults used to be kids too. To truly understand and relate to youth we have to be able to reflect on our own upbringing. Kids are kids and we should allow them to learn on their own with our guidance, support, and discipline. It's very important to never take their spirit away and understand that our words and actions have a direct impact on how a young athlete's mind-set develops in sports and in life. To truly understand the mind-set of a young athlete is to understand how we felt at their age. If you think your child or young athlete has a poor mind-set or attitude, then take a look at the influence you've impressed upon them.

2. The educational and instructional material the IYCA provides has helped me become the performance coach I am today. For all of us to be better, we need to constantly analyze our coaching style and techniques. We need to process information during training sessions and learn what motivates different athletes with different skill levels. Being conscious of the role parents play in the mind-set of our young athletes will help in the process of adapting our style for sending the appropriate message. Understanding the motivation and skill level of each athlete can help a performance coach learn if they need to delegate, inspire, guide, or direct their athletes to become better, mentally and physically.

3. Demanding respect as a parent, team coach, or performance coach is important for a young athlete to view us as role-models. Although kids are kids, they are very smart and can sense when we lose control – which leaves

room to question our authority. We have to be strong in our actions and words or they will never look up to us as role-models. We have to be strong leaders for guiding young athletes through adversity and consistent in our expectations, providing an environment for continual success, regardless of the circumstances.

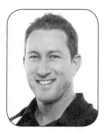

About Mike

Mike Pickles is well recognized in his community as an Athletic Performance Specialist and serves as the Head Strength & Conditioning Coach for The White Rock Titans Football organization. Mike is also the private Strength Coach for Ryan Williams, CPGA Pro on the Canadian Golf Tour, and helps prepare him during the off-season. He is the founder and president of 'myAthletic-Performance' Sport Specific Strength & Conditioning, specializing in long-term athletic development for youth in the South Surrey/White Rock area of British Columbia, Canada.

His athletic training facility is host to many local sports teams, giving young athletes the opportunity to develop the necessary skills to prepare them for long-term success in physical-fitness and sports. Mike is best known for his passion to bring the best out of his students through proper coaching and programming, making him the go-to-expert in his community.

Studying under some of the best Strength & Conditioning Coaches in world, Mike gives much credit to being a member of the International Youth Conditioning Association for providing excellent resources and support for his success. He holds a Diploma with a Declaration of Academic Achievement in Fitness & Health Promotion and is the recipient of the 2002 Health Systems Group Leadership Award.

Mike enjoys the West Coast lifestyle where he spends most of his free time golfing, hiking, mountain biking and snowboarding.

CHAPTER 4

A Coach's Opportunity to MAKE a Difference!

By Tom Hurley

NATHAN'S STORY

I was in the grocery store a while back, and ran into a former athlete of mine whom I had not seen since he graduated from High School in 2003. I was Nathan's soccer coach in seventh and eighth grade so it had actually been a dozen years since I had even spoken to him. I told him he had gotten tall; he told me I had gotten bald; typical "haven't seen you in ages" small talk. Our conversation ended a few minutes later with the usual "good to see ya, take care" and we began to continue with our shopping. As I turned to walk away, Nathan stopped me and said "Hey Mr. Hurley, I'm not sure if I ever took the time to thank you." I had no idea what he was talking about, however, the story that followed made me both extremely happy and a little sad at the same time.

Nathan explained to me that he knew that he was not a very good soccer player during the years that I had coached him. He knew that he was physically slow, lacked skill, and had a fairly limited knowledge of the game. He told me that he often wondered to himself why he was not cut from the team, or at the very least, kept from seeing any playing time. "After all" he said, "there were kids on that team who ended up winning a state championship and were on US National Teams." In no uncertain terms, Nathan was right. In every aspect of the sport, he was well behind other members of the team, except in one critical way – Nathan gave 100% of what he had to offer. Every minute of every practice, and every moment that he could spare, he remained positive and gave his best effort. And for this, he played in every game for two seasons in a row.

Nathan told me that, regardless of his lack of skill, he always strangely felt as though he belonged on that team, with that group of boys. He went on to say how difficult high school ended up being for him, and that he went through a lot of emotional turmoil during that time. He explained to me that during some of his lowest times, which actually included thoughts of suicide, he would take out his soccer mementos from seventh and eighth grade and that would help lift his spirits. More importantly, even though he was not your "typical athlete" and had stopped playing soccer, some of the friendships that he developed while on that team have remained to this day. I cannot relay all of what he told me during that short encounter, but suffice it to say as I stood there, there were moments when my heart hurt.

Nathan's little story left me speechless for a few awkward moments until I finally found myself saying, "you were treated with the same amount of care that everybody on that team was treated, no more, no less. You were kids; you wanted to play, so we played; simple. I never thought of any of you as soccer players, I thought of you as future husbands, and dads, and uncles, and co-workers, and at that moment in time, as twelve year-olds." And with that, Nathan thanked me once more and we parted ways.

Running into Nathan got me to thinking about the countless kids who don't get to experience sport this way; don't get to feel like they belong, get cut from programs without any other options available, get pressured to win, get treated like miniature adults by well-meaning coaches, and just end up quitting athletics or even physical activity altogether.

THE 1% RULE

In the course of a normal life of, say 80 years, the time most "athletes" spend in true competitive sport amounts to somewhere around 10% of their total life – usually between the ages of nine and seventeen. Some High School athletes will play in college, but most will not. That percentage is usually divided somewhat equally between hosts of coaches, in several sports, that most youth athletes will have during those years. A single coach's specific individual efforts are likely to encompass only about 1% of a child's entire life. Why then, do countless adults credit coaches that they had as children as having a lasting impact on their attitudes toward wellness, physical activity, and overall health?

Two critical psycho-social developmental stages occur during the exact time when most children begin competitive sport. The younger children, ages 7-11, are in the process of trying to figure out skills that they will carry with them for the rest of their lives. How to get along with peers, how to "belong," what it feels like to be socially accepted, the importance of personal friendship, realization of their own family dynamics as compared to their friends', and a true development of their own self-concept. The way that we encourage and include them at every opportunity fosters a healthy, long-lasting positive attitude toward activity, and bolsters a positive self-concept. Conversely, not being chosen as a "favorite" or being cut from teams with no other options to play available, sends a distinct negative message to that developing child.

Older athletes, ages 11-18, are smack dab in the middle of trying to find their own identity, constantly asking themselves, "Who am I?" They are seeking to establish who they are by reconsidering all of the goals and values set upon them by family and culture, including the culture of the sport(s) in which they are involved. It's the time in a young athlete's life when they need to hear that they are not defined by the sport that they play, rather that they are involved in a sport and that is a component of how they define themselves.

I have been coaching at one level or another on the youth scene for over thirty years. I have had the pleasure of training some exceptional groups and individuals who have wracked up some pretty impressive local, state, collegiate, national and international athletic honors. However whenever I get a chance to see a former athlete the conversation is less about sport than it is about what has happened in their lives since sport. We have an opportunity as coaches to leave an indelible positive mark on every athlete that we come in contact with.

SEVEN SIMPLE LETTERS

I hear it from coaches all of the time: "How are we supposed to make any kind of impact on a kid when we only get to see them twice a week for practice?" That sounds like a glass-half-empty way of looking at the situation. Why not say, "I get the chance to work with these kids twice a week, and I'm going to do my best to make a positive impact on them."

In a recent conversation I had with NFL Hall of Famer Joe De-Liemelleure, we got to talking about this very thing. I asked him what he remembered about his favorite youth coaches. "It wasn't about them, it was about the kids," he said. "They took the time to know all of us and didn't treat us all the same. They found out what made each of us tick." And most importantly "they reminded us that you don't go out and **work** football, you **play** football, or any sport for that matter."

In essence, it's all about how well you connect with each and every child you come in contact with. All of the most recent advances in fitness and training for youth can only be applied if indeed we are able to keep the youth involved in sport.

Here is a simple and effective way to make that happen:

CONNECT WITH YOUR PLAYERS

Care for your athletes

Objectivity is important

Needs of the child

Needs of the parent

Energy in your programming

Creativity in your programming

Time for play

Care about your athletes more than you care about the hardware. Trophies are nice; medals are cool, but in the long run they end up collecting dust just as easily as an old pair of socks in the corner. When members of your team know that you truly care about them as thinking, feeling people, well then you have something. As Joe D said, find out what 'makes them tick.' Treat them not as miniature adults, but as the age group that they are.

Objectivity is important when evaluating your players. Assumptions that one of your athletes will excel at a specific skill simply because a sibling of theirs did, or that they will enjoy a specific sport/position because they "have the build" for it, are unfair and often highly inaccurate. Become educated in both the art of coaching, and appropriate movement patterns for the particular developmental age group that you are coaching. Ask your organization's leadership to seek local experts to offer training. Many are willing to do this at little or no cost.

Needs of the child and **N**eeds of the parent are often out of synch with each other. This is a really tough one to address. I have coached teams in the past where on rare occasions parents have pulled their child from the program for a "more competitive" one, but moves like this often lead to disastrous results for the child. Be up front with the parents. Let them know what your intentions for their child are. I have found that an honest and direct dialogue with the parents has rarely let me down. As well, if the child understands that you and his/her parents have created this open dialogue, it lends credence to how much you care about them as individuals.

Energy in your programming cannot be understated. Let's face it, from a purely biological standpoint, young children were made to move and play. In the animal kingdom, it's how the young physically develop. Spending fifteen minutes to demonstrate a drill and expecting a nine year old to then go out and perform it with perfection is a recipe for failure. With younger athletes, keep the instructions short, and look for good movement. Don't get too technical. We've all seen youth soccer games that resemble a school of fish chasing around a piece of bread, and at some point, usually by accident, the ball ends up in the net. So what! There will be time to refine the game as they get older. The idea is to allow them to do what comes naturally, play.

Creativity in your programming can keep things fun. To this day I have my High School and Collegiate athletes do a crab-walk balloon breaking game as a warm-up activity for some fairly technical training sessions. Think back to your favorite games as a child and simply adapt them to your current sport. Allow your athletes time to come up with their own versions. Break out the Frisbees, Nerf balls, Hula Hoops, and use them in new ways. Believe me when I say this, from ages 7-21, none of my athletes look at these items the same way they used to!

Time for play is critical toward helping foster life-long activity. Ending a practice with sets of wind sprints is not only tedious, but can actually be counter-productive. How about a relay race? There is no question that the athletes are still sprinting, it's just more fun, and often the work to rest ratio makes a lot more sense. Tag games, challenge activities, relay races, even small-sided sport/game-type activities may be used. There is nothing better than seeing your team happy and tired after a practice. Joe D said it best when he shared, *"You don't work football, you play it."*

Take time to debrief the practice or game that you just ran your young athletes through. It's a really simple but invaluable tool in assessing your coaching/training success. All you need to do is run through the "CONNECT" checklist and give yourself a rating on each item. For example, think: "On a scale of 1-3 where one is the lowest score and three is the highest score, how would I rate myself on each of the items in the 'CONNECT' checklist?" Given that the needs of the kids and needs of the parents are combined, a self-score of 18 points would be 100%. Personally, I have never scored 18/18. There is always room for improvement. This is not a time to be self-critical, rather a time to recognize where adjustments need to be made.

THE 1% RULE REVISITED

I think about this often, the child that you impact today may not be a world leader, but all world leaders were children once. They were educated, loved, coached and cared for by a host of people who were once 1% of their lives. Be the coach that has a positive, lifelong impact on your athletes. After all, they will be moms and dads and quite possibly coaches themselves one day.

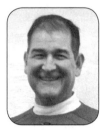

About Tom

Tom Hurley: M.Ed, CPT, YFS3, YNS, HSSCS, YSAS, is owner of Dominant Athletics, a performance-based training program for High School and Collegiate athletes, and *"Move Better, Play Better"* an athletic movement development program for athletes 7-13. He currently has programs with over 200 young athletes in individual, team, and club sports – from entry level to NCAA and Olympic Level competitors. Tom's unique education, firm grasp of child development and coaching theory, and extensive experience in counseling have made him highly sought out as a Mental Skills Coach as well.

Tom was classically trained in Health and Physical Education, earning his Bachelor of Science degree from Springfield College in 1983. His career path lead him to a large, private youth treatment facility where he eventually became a coordinator. As an individual and group therapist, he was recognized as a Masters Level Clinician by the State of New Jersey and coordinated several adolescent treatment facilities in that state. As his own family grew, Tom stepped out of that role and re-entered the educational field, first as a Lead Teacher for Public Alternative Education Program, then as a High School Health and Physical Education Teacher. Tom earned his M.Ed. from Wilkes University in Educational Development and Strategies, and has continued his education within the field of Sports Psychology at Argosy University.

Tom is currently Head of Youth Programming and Educational Development for Hangtime Fitness USA. Tom has enjoyed success in coaching several different sports at various levels. His youth teams have made it to state-level High School Post Season Tournaments in softball and soccer. His Boy's Soccer Team, of which he was the Assistant Coach, won the Pennsylvania State title in 2009.

CHAPTER 5

Fun and Fitness for 3 to 5-year-olds

Early adoption of fitness in a child's life will lay the foundation for youth athletic training.

By Jason Wong

I love fitness, I love training people and I've just recently figured out that I also love to teach. I've realized that even though I love to train youth athletes, I excel when it comes to teaching younger kids. I recently had a parent ask me if I had a teaching background. I told her that I didn't. She then asked how I learned to be so good working with children. I'm not quite sure, but if I had to guess I probably learned a lot being around my nieces and nephews. I love to play. I love sports. I like just messing around. My business partner and I are always trying a new challenge. One week it was throwing footballs into a mini basketball hoop on the other side of the facility. (For the record, I got mine in first!) Whatever it is that makes me good at working with kids, I am grateful because one thing I know is that you have to be good with kids if you want to teach them. There is a saying "You can't out train a bad diet." Well I'm telling you right now that, "You can't out program a bad coach." In other words, it doesn't matter if you have the best program in the world for 3 to 5-year-olds, or any age for that matter, if you aren't good with kids, find someone who is.

I constantly read books, emails, websites, articles, and magazines to further my knowledge. The fact that you are reading this book means you do the same. My goal is to help your work with 3 to 5-year-olds so that you will help them lay a foundation for youth athletic training.

Those of us who have kids know how important the first few years of a child's life are to their development. Every phase of a baby's development has a specific and important reason for preparing them for life. Our job as parents is to keep them safe and not interfere with what nature has intended to happen. Our job as coaches is pretty much the same: keep them safe and don't screw up their development.

Working with kids is pretty easy if you know what you are doing. Patience is a definite necessity. Understanding is probably even more important because you need to understand who you are teaching or training before you can actually teach or train them. Here's something that everyone knows, but no one remembers. Kids will do what you want them to do if you eliminate the other choices. For example I wanted to get my daughter off apple juice and decided I would let her drink grapefruit juice. Her options were water or grapefruit juice. After a few weeks of her telling me she didn't like grapefruit juice every time I gave it to her, she eventually started asking for it. The same goes with fitness. Kids will love movement and fitness if you take away the obstacles that prevent them from loving it.

I've come up with five principles that anyone who coaches this subset of kids needs to know. I call them my "Hi-5". Following them will make your life a whole lot easier. It will also help you achieve the results you are looking for from your kids.

1. TEACH DON'T TRAIN, PLAY DON'T TEACH

If you take nothing else away from the principles, *Teach Don't*

Train, Play Don't Teach is the most important because it is the cornerstone of any preadolescence class. Far too often coaches/parents get caught up in trying to train their kids when they should focus on playing with them and using these opportunities to teach them. The best part is that playing with some teaching is a whole lot easier than training. This is because the child is the one who teaches themselves. You are directing them, you are giving them an outlet to learn for themselves along with your guidance. If you don't think it makes sense think about your child's education. You don't train a kid to memorize every possible outcome to an addition problem, you teach them how to add. The same goes with athletic development. You don't train a kids to become an athlete first, you teach them to love movement (by playing), then playing sports, and then when their bodies are ready, you can train them in the art of athletics. If you think you can't teach your kids skills with out training them, you would be wrong. I have a class of (6-8) 3 to 5-year-olds. Almost all of them are skipping now, and all I did was ask them to skip (or gallop if they couldn't skip). I skip along with them so they can see what it looks like but that's pretty much it. After two weeks, my 3–year-old daughter was skipping by herself without me doing anything – except for staying out of her way and not providing unnecessary obstacles to her development. Kids learn by watching and doing. I'm not saying you can't correct stuff, but you have got to do it slowly. You can only cue one thing at a time with a child. If a child is trying to swing a bat and you tell them to switch hands, spread the feet, back elbow up, and watch the ball; the kid is just going to stare at you. They can't process that much information at one time, so stop trying to get them to do it. Teach kids, don't try and train them.

2. DO NOT DENY FITNESS

If at all possible, never deny a child fitness, make it as accessible as possible. That doesn't necessarily mean that you have to take them to the park everyday either. There are little things that children like to do that we adults tell them not to do. Case in point: My 3-year-old daughter was jumping on the couch the other day. I looked at her and told her to stop jumping on the couch because that is what we have been ingrained to tell children. I thought about it for a second and asked myself, "Why?" She's 3-years old she's not going to hurt the couch. We do have a fireplace with a stone hearth that she could hit if she jumped the wrong way, however that can easily be mitigated. So I walked over to her and I told her that she couldn't jump on the couch unless she asked me first. That way I am still in control of the behavior, she can't just do what she wants. Then I explained that she could only bounce in the middle but she could jump between the two as long as she was jumping away from the fireplace. She asked, "Why?" and I pointed to the fireplace and said I don't want you to jump/fall off and hit this because it would hurt. She looked at me and said, "I don't want to hit my head on that, okay daddy," kissed me and went on her way bouncing and laughing. There are many things we can do to let kids be kids, let them be active, but also keep them safe and obeying our rules. What can you do to let your child be more active?

3. LINK FUN TO FITNESS

To me this is the most interesting of the principles. I see so many programs that are all about fun, but very little fitness. Don't get me wrong, dancing and singing is great, but its a small part of a good program, not the entire program. Kids need to run, jump, climb, crawl, hit, kick, catch, and throw; all of which can be done in a fun manner. Your job is to make it happen. On the other end of the spectrum are the programs that are more training than anything else. For 3 to 5-year-olds, this is not appropriate and is borderline irresponsible. Fitness at this age group, if done properly, should be equal parts fun and fitness. Remember, little things make a big difference. Jumping on the couch, running down the sidewalk, and jumping up over cracks are all little things kids like to do that can keep them moving and linking fun to fitness. But there are so many other things you can do with 3 to 5-year-olds that will help them develop the way nature intended them to. Balloons are a fun tool/toy to teach kids how to kick, throw, and catch that you can use indoors without worrying about breaking something. Mix it up and have them try to only hit or kick with one side of their body, then try the other side. They won't always get it right and some of the kids that I teach at this age hardly ever get it right, but that's ok. Don't worry about the result, just focus on the process. Are they moving? Are they having fun? Are they learning? If so, that is all that matters at this point.

4. MOVE, MOVE, AND THEN MOVE SOME MORE

I think the first time I heard the term, 'Movement Must Dominate', it was from Brian Grasso, founder and former CEO of the IYCA. If you think about it, it's easy to see why. Name one sport where movement is not involved. Any youth program revolving around fitness or athleticism that does not incorporate all kinds of movement is a waste of time and a road block to your child's athletic development. My 3-year-old daughter loves to run around. When we go anywhere she is always running. To reference back to the Don't Deny Fitness principle, whenever we are out somewhere and she wants to run – as long as it is safe for her and any people that may be around – we play this game where she is allowed to run in front of us until my wife or I say "Stop." She cannot go anywhere until one of us walks up to her and taps her on the head. Then she takes off again. This ensures that she gets to run, but also she doesn't get too far in front of us. Simple games like this lead me into my next principle.

5. REWARD THE BEHAVIOR, NOT THE OUTCOME

This is often the most misunderstood principle. You have to remember at this age we are trying to get the kids to like fitness and movement. If your child doesn't like movement, they will not be a very good athlete, its pretty simple. By focusing on rewarding the behavior, we are encouraging children to continue that behavior, which in our case is movement. I'm not saying to that you cannot reward the outcome, but you need to focus on rewarding the behavior as well. I have a couple kids in my classes that are not as advanced as the others, so if all I did was reward the outcome, these kids would never get a "win." Every child needs to have a win here and there. By win, I mean a success, something that they succeeded in doing that acknowledges their effort. "Good Job Billy!! You're went way farther in your bear crawl today than you did last week!!" means nothing to us, but may be the difference from this child buying into what you are teaching or not wanting to attend anymore.

These five principles, although written with the 3 to 5-year-old in mind, also works with older children. I use these same 5 principles with all my classes, which run up to 13 years old. I often get asked if we have other classes that are more aggressive or in depth... (yes, parents of 3 to 5-year-olds ask that!) It's not their fault though, they have been conditioned to believe that if some is good more is better. With kids, that could not be farther from the truth and guess what - all the science backs you up. I have yet to read an article that espouses the benefits of upping the training intensity for children, however I have read several articles that emphasize the risks associated with over-training or sports-specific training.

There you have it, the 5 principles that you need to use when dealing with 3 to 5-year-olds. Remember, when its comes to kids, relax a bit, have fun, and enjoy knowing that you are making a huge difference in their lives.

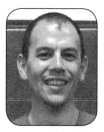

About Jason

Jason Wong is the Founder and Director of Youth Fitness of Red Zone Training, The San Ramon Valley's Premier Youth Fitness Facility. Teaching and coaching has become his passion, but he does not claim to have all the answers so he is constantly studying. "If I'm not teaching/coaching/training, and that is the order they should be in, I'm studying and learning." He primarily works with 3 to 13-year-olds of all fitness levels.

Jason believes that coaches who work with kids would be better served by learning more about working with children instead of spending all their time learning about the newest must-have training device/program. He also recommends that coaches follow the 'less is more' approach when dealing with kids.

Jason is a National Strength and Conditioning Association Certified Personal Trainer, as well as a Level 3 Youth Fitness Specialist and a High School Strength and Condition certification holder through the International Youth Conditioning Association.

CHAPTER 6

My STORY
Road To Success

By Anthony Hart Trucks

Click! That was the sound of the seatbelt locking into place when I was three years old and I was in the front seat looking back at my three younger half-siblings. We were all being sent off to foster homes because my biological mom called social services and said she could no longer take care of her children. I was the oldest, with no biological father in sight and my younger siblings all had the same father, but he wasn't in the picture either. For the next three years of my life I would be bouncing around the east Contra Costa county of the San Francisco Bay area between multiple foster homes – with no knowledge of what my future might be from one day to the next. I remember homes where I would be deprived of food, and my only meal of the day would be a small fry from a nearby burger joint. I would be forced to ride in a shopping cart as it was pushed down a hill repeatedly against my wishes. I would be made to sit on the curb and forced to lick the bottom of the neighborhood kids shoes one by one, and the list could go on and on. I remember one home where the family I was living with for the week simply wanted to try out having a foster child, and it just so happened to be the week before they were headed to Disneyland for the weekend. So on that day, everyone got packed up and ready to leave, including myself, and they loaded up into their family van, and as I was getting in, I was told I was getting into the wrong car. I turned to see the social worker's car there, ready to take me to the next home. Let's just say continuity was something I had no experience with. My childhood was ridden with insecurity and a lack of any acceptance from even my very own mother, not to mention I had no idea where my siblings were placed either.

At six years of age, I was driven to a home in Antioch, California. This would be the final stop on my wild ride of foster homes, but by no means was the roller coaster that I would call my life, pulling into the starting gate anytime soon. I was brought to a home where I showed up in flooding purple corduroys and black boots that were too small for my feet. This was due to the fact that some foster children are looked at as a paycheck instead of as a child. I was now the lone African-American in an all-white family. I was instantly accepted by this family and life moved forward. This new family was by no means 'picture perfect' and in the simplest words I can put it in, we were as dysfunctional as they come. Across the board, not just to me, there was physical abuse, emotional abuse, poverty, and so much more. Basically, life didn't pick up and get better, it simply was different for me. For the next eight years of my life, I experienced some of the highest highs of my life and some pretty low lows. One of the major problems I faced was the fact that my biological mother still had parental rights, even though she did not live with me. This caused me to be unable to play sports or take trips, because she wouldn't allow it simply out of spite for the family, because she blamed her problems on them, oddly enough, as if it was their fault that I was in foster care. She would also torment me by telling me to wait by the window and she would come in the night to get me, and I remember night after night crying myself to sleep waiting for her and her never coming. The list of her torment was endless, it seems, but at 14 years old, I stood in front of her in court and pleaded with the courts to have her rights severed, and I was finally adopted by this new family, legally. Life began anew for me.

The next years of my life would be littered with hardships as well as high points. My adoptive Mom, Gina, was diagnosed with MS. I sucked at sports for the first two years I played. My adoptive brother almost died. I was offered a scholarship to play football in college. I accepted Jesus Christ as my Lord and savior. I met a girl in high school that I eventually would go on to marry. I was homecoming king. My biological family came out of the woodwork when I went to college. My adoptive grandfather committed suicide. My high school girlfriend attended college with me; I had my first son in college at 20 years old with no support but my girlfriend, and I stayed beyond faithful to her and we stuck it out together. My eventual wife helped me find my biological father, who I found out had no idea I existed. I met my father and his side of the family during my first college start ever in Mississippi and we won. I tore my shoulder playing football. I entered the NFL draft and was signed as a PFA. I got married and my wife graduated *summa cum laude* with her masters in four years; I went on to play with the Buccaneers, Redskins, and Steelers. I graduated from college with a degree focused in biology anatomy and human physiology. I tore my other shoulder; I came home and opened a gym where I could provide a world-class training experience, because I absolutely love training people. I had twins who are now two, and the list is missing a lot, but could go on and on. Which brings me to today – happy, healthy and STILL standing.

MY PLAYING DAYS

The first two years of me playing sports I was horrible, to say the least, mostly because I was years behind my peers, because I was now 14 and just finally starting to play sports. I heard things like, "butter fingers," "you're slow," "you suck," and I'm sure you get the picture. It was at this point that I had to take a good look at myself and decide who I wanted to be, the kid who went through a lot as a child and was ready to say 'enough is enough' and give up, or the kid who went through a lot, and was going to be an example to the world that I had what it took to be successful. Where you start doesn't determine where you finish, its WHERE YOU FINISH that matters! I spent the next off-season tirelessly preparing both my mind and body to outdo what even I thought I was capable of doing. A day LITER-ALLY never went by that I wasn't holding onto a football, or at the local park running routes alone or with a friend. Needless to say, I was determined to accomplish more than anyone thought I could, and the hardest part was not trying to convince others that I could be better, it was convincing MYSELF, because all my life I had been told and shown by the world that I was worthless to them. If I believe in me, then everyone else will eventually follow, but only if my resolve was tireless – and it was by every sense of the word both in my words AND my actions.

The following year, a monster arrived at pre-season football training and he never left. This athlete was not only better physically prepared, but he was beyond mentally prepared. Only I knew how much work and effort I put into preparing for that season, and I never wanted to "tell" people this fact, I wanted them to experience it for themselves and let the words pass through their lips on their own, "what did HE do in the offseason?" I was faster than everyone on the team, I was quicker, I was stronger, and boy was I mean. This was my opportunity to show the world that I was NOT worthless. I had always been the outcast, the "white washed" black kid who didn't fit in with the other black kids, and I was black, so I didn't always fit in with the white kids. I was the odd man out until I hit that football field; it was there that I MORE than fit in, I set the curve. Nowhere else had I ever FELT the amount of freedom and acceptance in my life, and it became my drug. It was my way to escape the cruel world that I seemed to have been placed in, and I could create my own world, free of the life that seemed to have been written for me. "I" finally had control of something in my life for the first time. The most integral part of this new change was my attitude on every play. Because I had gone through so much and still worked so hard to prepare, I would never quit, ever. The harder I worked, the harder it was to EVER quit.

From there I went on to earn a football scholarship to the University of Oregon, where I played as a true freshman and started my true sophomore year over a senior. I then went on to become a standout player, and in my senior year I led the Pac-10 conference in sacks, tackles- for-loss, forced fumbles, fumbles recovered, and was 6th in total tackles, even while missing a whole game. I also went on to be co-defensive MVP of the Holiday Bowl even though we lost, because I had such a good game against Adrian Peterson and the Oklahoma Sooners. I went on to play in the NFL for the Tampa Bay Buccaneers under coach Jon Gruden, the Redskins under Joe Gibbs, and the eventual 2008 Super Bowl Winning Pittsburgh Steelers under coach Tomlin. Sadly, I tore my shoulder in the first preseason game of 2008 against the Eagles, and it ended my season, …and eventually my career. My playing days came to a close, but my burning desire to accomplish more than the world ever thought I could just took a new turn, and kept on pushing forward. My effort never stopped, it just refocused and the direction it went in was what I feel is my true calling. I now get to give back to other people in a way that was never done for me. I am now the change I want to see in the world.

HANGING UP THE JERSEY

When my career came to a close, it was time to move forward with life because I now had a wife, 3 children, and bills to pay, because life doesn't simply slow down when you want it to; so you can complain because it just got harder or you can pick yourself up and show the world it can't keep you down. Moving on was hard on my heart, and I needed to fill a gap left by my inability to play. That gap was filled by my dormant dream to train others. I had always wanted to open a gym and train others, and I had received my degree in that area for that purpose. It was now time to pursue that dream. I had some money in the bank, a dream, passion, and what I feel was God's voice saying to me, "Son, it's time." So I jumped in 'full bore' with everything I had.

Sadly, I had no idea how to run a business, and in November of 2010, I almost lost my gym. My love of training has carried me so far because I absolutely love what I do, which allows my clients to not only get results physically, but they get the mental push they need as well, because I bring every bit of my bubbling personality out so that they have a phenomenal experience. I want to give every client I have an experience far greater than I could have ever wished I could have had, and more. On the flip side, without business knowledge, I was doomed to fail. So again I had a major turning point in my life and I had to dig in and give it my all to succeed. Let's just say I was able to do it again. I am still here and prospering and I am happier than I ever have been. I love simply stopping and looking at what I have been able to accomplish because I failed to give in. I have a beautiful wife, healthy children, my wife owns a business, I have two great families, and I have a gym and gym family that was started from scratch. It includes so many awesome people and experiences to date. My football career ended so that my life career could begin.

LIFE LESSONS LEARNED THROUGH SPORTS

In all of this, I am sure you're wondering what this has to do with sports, and more importantly, with you. The answer is everything. My experiences as a child and an athlete are a way to show you that life and sports go hand in hand. In life, many of us play the outcast role, and it's hard to become "part" of something; then you join a sports team and again you become the outcast simply looking to become "part" of the team. In life and in sports you're always trying to figure out where you belong, because it's important to 'belong" to something in life, as it's our human nature to be around other people and develop meaningful relationships. In life and sports there are bumps along the road, be it troubles in life that are out of our control or injuries in sports that are out of our control. There are so many things in both arenas that relate to each other, and I personally feel that all life's lessons can be found within the sports world and can be applied to the "real" world.

Determination, Work Ethic, Perseverance, Teamwork, and a slew of other life traits can all be learned through finding something that you don't do well and doing everything in your power to make yourself better at it, no matter what stands in your way. You must be relentless and tireless in your pursuit of accomplishing you goal, or you stand to lose out on "what could have been" …because the path to hell is paved with good intentions! So you MUST see everything to the very end, and not just start something. It's like having faith, I don't mean religious faith. I mean faith in the fact that with hard work you BELIEVE anything can happen. Without it nothing has ever been accomplished that is worthwhile, and I personally can attest to this. No one can show you or tell you that you can't accomplish anything that you want, because they aren't YOU. Truth is, nothing in this world will ever be handed to you, so if YOU don't go grab it, you will NEVER attain it. *So you should never even start to listen to other people tell you what you can or can't do with yourself.* Most importantly, it teaches you the importance of teamwork, and in my case, family. Without that "family" atmosphere, you stand to gain nothing in life that will have any meaning for you. You absolutely need that support, which is why I base all that I do around my family both at home and at work, because it is the driving force of the human race. In essence, learn to master the world of sports as an athlete whether you are the star or not, and you will learn invaluable life skills that can take you to places you only pictured in your "dreams," because it's not about being the best out there at what you do. Its about being the best YOU that you can put out there. Live a life worth telling about, because no one wants to hear the stories of a person who "almost" made something of themselves.

Tough times don't last forever, tough people do – because the human will to succeed is directly proportional to the will to never quit, and the harder you work the harder it IS to quit. There are two types of people in this world, those that work, and those that watch them at work. I don't mind the audience.

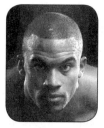

About Anthony

Anthony Trucks, B.S., C.S.C.S. Owner, Founder, Director of Trucks Training Inc. graduated from Antioch High School in 2002 where he started his career in sports. Anthony endured a lot at a young age and made it his life's goal to overcome obstacles that others would say he was incapable of. Even in high school he took the extra time to train on his own to achieve his highest possible physical level. Anthony's hard work paid off and he earned a football scholarship to the University of Oregon. In his time there, he decided that whatever his future was, he wanted it to include a future in training other individuals to reach their highest level of physical goals attainable. For this reason, he decided to work towards a Bachelors of Science with focuses in Human Anatomy, Biology, and Human Physiology.

During his time at Oregon, he made sure to pay close attention to the training he was doing and especially "why" he was performing the specific exercises and programs. By doing this, he was able to get better every year and perform better on the field. He started as an outside linebacker his true sophomore year and played well. His senior year he led the Pacific 10 Conference in sacks, tackles for loss, forced fumbles, fumbles recovered, and was 5th in total tackles. He was also the Co-Defensive MVP of the 2005 Pacific Life Holiday Bowl even though his team lost.

He participated in the 2006 NFL Combine and was signed by the Tampa Bay Buccaneers as a free agent in March of 2006. He has played with the Washington Redskins and the Pittsburgh Steelers since. He then suffered a season-ending left shoulder injury in the first pre-season game of the 2008 NFL season. Throughout his entire college and NFL career, Anthony collected invaluable information on ways to make himself better, which he translates into making others better! When his NFL playing days came to a close, his goal was to make others better than he ever was.

Anthony has been progressing towards building his career post football since he started college. He has since achieved a personal training certification from the National Council on Strength and Fitness, as well as his certification as an NSCA-Certified Strength and Conditioning Specialist. Anthony's main goal is to lose the stereotypical label of athletes turned coaches being poor coaches. For that reason, Anthony spends countless hour LEARNING and mastering his craft so that he could harbor as much knowledge as others in the industry, while still having been blessed enough to play his sport at the highest level in the world. So Anthony's clients can trust they are getting the same quality training as the professionals they admire. Anthony can be reached at Trucks Training at 925-756-7321 or through his website at: www.TrucksTraining.com.

CHAPTER 7

Athletic Specific Fitness
Athlete First, Sports Player Second

Mike Barone, NSCA-CPT

Unfortunately, with the politics and competitive nature of youth athletics today, the emphasis on technical skill and game experience has made developing athletes, instead of sport players, unbalanced. The goal of the athlete, regardless of his or her chosen sport, should be to become the best athlete that he or she can possibly be. Developing athleticism will pay the athlete dividends not only for his or her sport seasons, but for a lifetime. In my opinion, coaching the well-rounded athlete versus the technically-sound player is more desirable, because they are more apt to learn, can adapt more easily, and are less prone to injury. Therefore, the focus should be on athleticism first, and sport technical skills second.

Some common problems I notice within the preparation for youth athletics are: too much emphasis on wins and losses and sport technique, and not enough emphasis on athletic development. In addition, there are coaches, parents and young athletes who lack the knowledge of developing sound athleticism, indicating the need for proper coaching from qualified trainers or performance coaches. There are athletes who play one sport exclusively; run long distance and do some token push-ups and sit-ups for conditioning; maintain the "more is better" syndrome with an imbalanced focus on intensity; have the weight-room mentality of, "How big and strong can I get?" and hit the weight room haphazardly, without a plan or understanding of why or what to do. Instead you need to adopt an athletic mentality of "How can I become the best athlete I can possibly be?" and focus on development and progress through movement-based training (athletic fitness).

Regardless of sport or not, you are more an athlete than a body builder, so training in the gym should not be isolated muscle-group training only. Your training should actually bridge the gap between the weight room and the field of play. Essentially, it is all about developing athleticism and enhancing performance, and not how much weight you can lift in the gym! So, you can't go wrong if you focus on training movements, not muscles. We all have a need to move; some may move faster and more fluidly than others, but our bodies need to locomote, push/pull, lower and raise our center of mass, and rotate – in order to function. Below you will find some examples of the 4 Pillars (categories) of Movement that all training should include in order to develop an efficient usable body.

CATEGORIES OF MOVEMENT – 4 PILLARS	
PUSH-PULL	STANDING & LOCOMOTION
Standing Band Press Push-ups Standing Band Pulls Band archer pulls	1 leg anterior reaches 1 leg body weight squats 1 leg Romanian Dead Lifts
LEVEL CHANGE	ROTATION
Prisoner Squats Split Squats Lunges	Medicine ball twists Pulls with rotation i.e. Archer Pulls T-Stabilization push-ups

SPORT SPECIFIC OR ATHLETE SPECIFIC?

As a trainer I hear all too often when parents come in looking for training for their son or daughter, "Will the training be sports specific (i.e. for soccer or baseball etc.)?" In most cases my response is that the training will be athletic specific, not necessarily sports specific. That said, there will be some specific movements or protocols that will address the demands at their given sport, however the bulk of the training is about athletic enhancement in which the focus is on improving the qualities that will make them a well-rounded athletic individual. This will enable him or her to take those qualities and apply them to the skills and technical work that they do in practice to enhance their overall performance in that sport. *We need to develop an athlete first and a sports player second.* When we develop the athlete first, he or she can become a player of any sport because the athletic foundation is strong. The athletic qualities and development will pay greater dividends for a lifetime. With my youth athletes, my goal is to make them move the best that they can, and to make them get better, stay healthy, and instill lifetime habits of fitness and function. Training athletically will make them stronger, more agile, and have more body control. They will also be more mobile, flexible, and better conditioned.

Athletic Qualities Desired
- Speed
- Strength
- Power
- Stability
- Agility
- Balance
- Coordination
- Rhythm
- Timing
- Reaction

IS THERE A NEED FOR SAFE, EFFECTIVE AND APPROPRIATE TRAINING FOR YOUTH ATHLETES?

I had the opportunity to sit in on a U12 girls' soccer program as their coaches were putting them through a fitness/training session indoors. They were utilizing a college gymnasium and a weight room. The gymnasium session consisted of different stations for the group of girls to go through in a circuit-type fashion until all stations were complete one time through. The format was appropriate for the large group, but what was not so appropriate was the exercise selections, the complexity of them, the lack of progression, and quality of coaching for safety and progressive results. Next, two of the coaches brought a group of girls into the weight room to do circuit strength training. The problem was they had just completed the circuit in the gymnasium and were fatigued. They were instructed to use the machines and once again the coaches lacked the knowledge of what was appropriate and what proper progression might look like. The coach had one little girl try to do a standing military press in a Smith machine – which is a bar that travels in a fixed, straight up and down path and the bar alone weighs 45lbs. The girl couldn't maintain a strong and stable core and was arching while struggling to lift the bar. To another girl, the coach told her that she needed to lie on the hamstring curl machine and do curls because her hamstrings weren't as strong as her quads. Both examples of a well-meaning coach with a little bit of knowledge that makes them dangerous. I left shaking my head.

ARE MACHINES A GOOD FIT FOR YOUTH ATHLETES?

One of my former clients was a 10-year-old tennis player. At the second session I had with this athlete, he brought me a note from his mom stating that I needed to implement what his previous trainer did, including adapting the leg extension machine so that he could use it to strengthen his knees because they bothered him after tournaments. I wouldn't put most adults, including myself, on that machine, and especially not a very small, 10-year-old athlete. Also, the athlete's knees didn't hurt because they were weak; they hurt because of overuse in his sport due to sport specialization and his previous trainer's lack of knowledge to assist the proper development of this youth athlete. There were two problems here, an overzealous mom with good intentions, and a trainer that really did this young athlete a disservice – by trying to fit him into an adult machine that had no purpose in his athletic development or his structural health. This is an example of why we can't and shouldn't make young athletes mini-adults.

DOES GOING TO THE GYM GUARANTEE RESULTS?

On paper, going to the gym 2-3 times a week along with sport practice may look like dedication, but if you're not getting anything accomplished while you're there or you don't have a well-developed plan, you are only wasting your time, and quite possibly doing more harm than good. I hear a lot from some of the high school athletes that I train that the coach has mandatory weight-room two times a week. It will either be some program they took out of an old school book or magazine, or they just have to show up and check in – which ends up being a social hour with a few sets of bench press, arms, and a lot of sit-ups.

To be the best athlete you can be, these six areas must be addressed in your training:
1. Functional/Athletic Strength training – training movements not muscles (address the 4 pillars of movement)

2. Core strength and stability

3. Mobility and flexibility

4. Power

5. Metabolic Conditioning – circuits, intervals (endurance)

6. Recovery and regeneration - Foam roll, stretching

Utilizing these six areas within your training will pay great dividends. Through preparation you will gain confidence, move better and more efficiently, gain better body control, as well as be better conditioned. Your balance, stability, strength, and power will improve. Additional benefits include improved rhythm, timing and reaction, along with increased mobility and flexibility. You will enhance your ability to recover and reduce the occurrence of injuries. Now let's get started! Below is your guide to enhanced athleticism.

Ways to Train:
- Standing 90-95% of time
- Single Leg
- Explosive / Dynamic
- 3-Dimensional (multi-planar)
- Movements not muscles
- Integrated / Total Body
- Balance / Stability
- Rotational
- Foam Roll - Dynamic Warm-up or Movement Prep / Joint Mobility

Address each of the 4 pillars of movement in your workouts – locomotion, push/pull, level changes and rotation

Use Proper Progression:
- Learn before you intensify
- Slow to Fast
- Easy to Hard
- Body weight before external resistance
- Stable to unstable
- Simple to complex
- Regress to progress if needed

Equipment/Tools to Utilize:
- ✔ Body weight
- ✔ Medicine Balls
- ✔ Bands / Pulleys
- ✔ Stability Balls
- ✔ Kettlebells
- ✔ Dumbbells
- ✔ Jump Ropes
- ✔ Heavy Ropes

- ✔ Agility Ladders
- ✔ Suspension Trainer / TRX
- ✔ Foam Rollers
- ✔ Dyna Disc / Disc Pillow
- ✔ Airex Pad

With the proper coaching and the right tools, you can get a great workout almost anywhere. (*For all of your training and workout equipment needs, visit: www.performbetter.com.)

Here are some examples of a transition from a typical gym-type workout to an athletic-type (more functional) workout.

GYM WORKOUT VS. ATHLETIC WORKOUT	
NOT THIS (Machines, Isolated Body Part Training)	**THIS** (Integrated Movement Training)
Treadmill – warm-up and stretch	Foam Roll – Dynamic Warm-up or movement prep
Leg Extension	1 Leg Body Weight Squat
Leg Curl	Stability Ball Leg Curl or 1 leg RDL (stiff leg dead lift)
Bench Press	Standing Band Press or Push-ups
Seated Row	Standing Band Pull or Band Archer Pull
Seated Dumbbell Press Biceps Curls Triceps Extension	Standing Kettlebell Curl, Press, Overhead Extension
Abs Machine or Crunches	TRX Knee Tucks or Medicine Ball Diagonal Wood Chops

SAMPLE CIRCUIT WORKOUT

Implement using time (30 seconds on, 15 seconds off) or by counting reps, completing one to three rounds of each circuit with a two-minute rest period between each circuit.

Circuit 1:

1. BW 1 leg anterior reach
2. BW push-ups
3. TRX reclined pull-up
4. MB twist

REST PERIOD – 2 minutes

Circuit 2:

1. Band step press (opposite arm, opposite leg)
2. Band step pull (using two hands)
3. Dumbbell lateral reaching lunges
4. MB side bends

REST PERIOD – 2 minutes

Circuit 3:

1. MB reverse lunge with rotation
2. 1 leg dumbbell alternating curl & press
3. Band archer pulls
4. SB Knee tucks

(BW=Body Weight; TRX=Suspension Trainer; MB=Medicine Ball; SB=Stability Ball) Improved strength, conditioning, flexibility, mobility, enhanced movement and athleticism, all rolled up in one.

IN SUMMARY

If you set out to enhance your athleticism and train for an athletic, usable body; one that has 'giddy up' behind the physique, you're going to need a purposeful program. You will need to have a focused goal in mind and have a good "why" for the type of training you will do. Your purpose needs to make sense for what you are trying to accomplish (enhanced athleticism) and needs to be balanced (not just certain body parts). Your training needs to resemble athletic movement.

Our muscles must work in concert in order for the body to work as a unit.

Remember, just like the saying "there is no 'I' in TEAM because Together Everyone Achieves More" That is how the muscles in your body work – TOGETHER (collectively) – and for that to happen you'll need to train the body as a unit by training movements, not muscles. So, train outside of your sport for your sport, ditch the machines, get focused and have a plan, and train purposefully, functionally and athletically!

Mike Barone, NSCA-CPT
Rochester, NY
Dynamic Function, Inc.
www.dynamicfunction.com

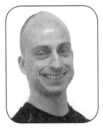

About Mike

Mike Barone, owner of Dynamic Function, Inc., is a fitness industry veteran since 1989 and has been working as a Personal Trainer since 1991. Mike has trained numerous athletes at the youth, high school, college and professional levels. He served as the Strength and Conditioning Coach for the 2002 Monroe Community College Men's Soccer Team, and the 2003, 2004, and 2010 Rochester Raging Rhinos Professional Soccer Team.

Mike is certified with the NSCA and NASM as a Personal Trainer, and with the USA Track & Field as a Level 1 Coach. Mike is also a Certified American Kettlebell Club Coach and an Art of Strength Certified Kettlebell Trainer.

CHAPTER 8

Parents Guide To Developing The Talented Athlete

By Wendy Breault

If you are a parent interested in what it takes to help your child develop into a talented athlete, it might be safe to say that you yourself might have a touch of drive, passion and competitiveness. I'm going to warn you that the content of this chapter may be frustrating for you! Why? Because there are no offerings of immediate drills, training or exercises to do in the backyard or at the gym that will turn your child into a talented athlete. What this chapter divulges is that it is the slow, methodical process of training over the long haul that will eventually give your son or daughter the biggest advantages. For most parents this means putting on the brakes.

Developing the talented athlete takes patience and discipline on the parts of the adults and programs that are training them. It requires the use of sound, evidence-based practices, long- term planning and an integrated systematic approach. Unfortunately, in comparison to other countries, the United States has yet to show interest in developing any kind of integrated system. Many countries including Canada, Britain, Australia and New Zealand are in process of developing comprehensive, integrated approaches to training their youth in physical fitness and sports. Basing their programs on sound up to date science, these countries are all using similar forms of long-term athletic development. In fact, in recognizing the effectiveness of the long-term approach, many have identified such programs as a way of cultivating elite talent for their Olympic Programs.

There is a wealth of scientific information on youth athletic development; however, in the United States, it seems to rarely be used as a basis for the development of youth training programs. As parents, we see no coordinated efforts, no integration between entities such as schools, sports associations, traveling clubs or training facilities. Children are therefore over trained, trained inconsistently and trained in accordance to what the program's needs are, rather than that of the child's best interests. There are no standard requirements for athletic programs and rarely are there any requirements regarding coach education, training, certifications or licensing. Because of this, for parents, finding quality sports programs and coaching can be a really a difficult process.

In order to be able to be a smart "consumer" and really to ensure your child's safety, emotional well-being and the ability to reach optimal athletic potential, you need to familiarize yourself with what sound athletic development practices look like. The following is a description of one of the important concepts regarding children's athletic development, the fact that it is a long- term process in which there exist shorter critical windows of opportunity or periods of "trainability." Provided is a short discussion of the athletic model Canada presently is using, Long Term Athletic Development or LTAD. A shortened list of LTAD stages is outlined to show how skills and training approaches are built progressively. Furthermore a list of suggested guidelines is provided to assist parents in finding good athletic training services for their children.

A number of scientists have found that there are critical times during a child's development – where their system is primed for acquiring specific movement patterns and skills. It has been demonstrated that exposing children to the right skills at the right times maximizes their athletic development. Each set of athletic skills or movement patterns is a building block for the next and need to be obtained in progressive order. The ability of the athlete to perform technically sophisticated sport skill is completely dependent on the acquisition of early fundamental skills during their critical developmental period.

Scientist Istvan Balyi used these principles in developing the framework for the Long Term Athletic Development Model. Balyi's LTAD is a model based on human growth and development, it is meant to provide an optimal blueprint for training and developing athletes to their full potential. Balyi refers to the critical developmental periods as "windows of opportunity."

Not learning a skill during the critical period or missing the "window of opportunity" makes it much harder and may altogether hinder the ability to fully acquire a skill. A great example of an "intellectual" window of opportunity is the natural ability for toddlers and young children when exposed, to fully master multiple languages. In contrast, it becomes more difficult as children get older to learn other languages, and for adults even more so, if not impossible to fully acquire fluent skills. The same holds true for athletic windows of opportunities. Balyi has found that the most important times or critical periods for acquiring athletic skill are pre –pubescent, during, and just after the peaks of children's growth spurts. He has pointed out that during these times, children obtain the foundation for most all of their later athletic abilities. He has found that missing skills during these windows results in permanent deficiencies in athletic ability.

How does one miss a window of opportunity? Well, through the absence of exposure. Again the child learns the language because he or she is exposed to it in the environment. Maybe some guidance, but really little instruction is needed, for the child to "pick up" the language. In the same way, a child will pick up physical skill as long as they are challenged and given plenty of opportunities to experiment and practice it. A parent or coach cannot always know when kids are at their peak for critical periods, so, the best way to help your child develop skills and lay down the early building blocks, is simply to expose them to as much of a variety of physical challenges and sports as possible. The more they are exposed to multiple physical challenges at young ages, the more likely they are to absorb or pick up the right skills at the right times.

Balyi's LTAD model outlines the following stages for when children experience windows of opportunity and are most ready to learn skills. Chronological ages are listed, however the true model uses a formula to measure developmental stages according to growth spurts. The stages are named *Fundamentals, Learning to Train, Training to Train, Training to Compete* and *Training to Win.*

The *Fundamental* period is between the ages of 6 and 8 for girls and 7 and 9 for boys. This is a window of opportunity for developing speed and agility; it is also essential that the following fundamental skills are learned in this period as they are the foundation for all athletic movement: running, jumping, throwing, kicking, catching and swimming. It is very important that the child is introduced to physical activity in fun ways, and finds exercise enjoyable. This lays the foundation of experiencing sports as life-long enjoyable activities. Variety is the key to your child developing all around athletic ability.

Learn to Train is the stage that identifies the time span at the approximate ages of 9-12 for boys and 8-11 for girls. During this time is an optimal window for skill training and developing physical literacy (competence in fundamental movement and sports skills that are the foundation for all sports). Children should be starting to show some mastery over the fundamental movement skills, and will generally begin to show some interest and ability to learning basic sports skills. Again, exposure to a variety of sports is more beneficial to the athlete's success than specializing in one sport.

Train to Train is around the approximate ages of 12-16 for boys and 11-15 for girls. Important windows of opportunity during these years are strength, endurance and speed. During this time, athletes should also begin to work more on, and gain more, specific technical sport skills.

Train to Compete is identified as the time of about 15 or 16. This stage is meant to guide the training regimen of the athlete who is intent on competing at high levels. It is at this point the competitive athlete really begins to focus all their attention and specializes in his or her sport. They should by this time be proficient in all basic movement patterns and in their sports-specific movements patterns and are able to apply their skills to intense competitive environments. Training is mostly technical preparation with more focus on competition.

Train to Win – Age 19 and up. This is the elite stage of development, where athletes are completely focused on sports preparation and competition with the purpose of winning in mind.

Please notice that these stages start at early childhood and go through to adulthood. This is because it takes from early childhood to adulthood to develop the talented athlete. It is a long-term process. You must have patience in allowing development to occur as nature intended. If you as a parent rush this process, or allow a coach to push training and skills onto your child prior to their body's ability to adapt functionally, you and/or the coach will have interfered with your child's ability to reach their full athletic potential. Your child will be at risk for injury and burnout, and with repeated acceleration of training, will peak in their performance far earlier in their development. This premature peaking impedes the athlete from ever reaching their true potential. The important message here is to expose your child to sports and activities, not *impose*. Find a coach or program that both understands and follows the guiding principles of long-term athletic development.

HERE ARE SOME GUIDELINES THAT CAN HELP YOU NURTURE YOUR DEVELOPING ATHLETE

As a parent, you must educate yourself so that you know what to look for and be able to recognize components of a good program. Beware of becoming drawn into programs making big promises of gains in short periods of time, programs that point to either their being college or professional athletes or training college or professional athletes as being a qualification for working with your child. Or programs that point towards high buck flashy training equipment as the secret to their athlete's success. Good programs will produce and work with good athletes, they may utilize certain pieces of equipment, and they themselves may be well-respected athletes, it's just that one does not make the other. A good program will discuss their intent on contributing to the long-term success of your child. Though they may offer services in short segments, six weeks, 3 months etc. , they should be discussing the gains your child will be making in terms of sports season, multi-seasons or years. When asking programs for references or for examples of their athletes' accomplishments, ask about the athletes that have been with them over several years, not several months. This will be more indicative of their ability to develop athletes.

Again, expose your child to a wide variety of athletic activities and sports. The more exposure he or she has, the greater his or her chances are at acquiring fundamental movement patterns. Programs and coaches working with pre-pubescent children should be aware of the developmental windows and the skill-needs of the children they are coaching.

Don't push your young child or allow any coach or program to push them into focusing intensely on any one sport. (Exception to this rule is a sport such as gymnastics, where the highest level of competition peaks, in general, prior to the age of 18). Explain to your child that in order to become a really good baseball player, volleyball player, etc., you should play basketball and soccer and other sports. As they become more focused in their mid-teens, it becomes more appropriate for them to begin to concentrate in and utilize year-round training in one or two sports.

Be careful of programs and coaches that pride themselves in coaching advanced skills to young developing athletes. Children should always be allowed to challenge themselves and try new things; however, forcing technical skills prior to their ability to master them ultimately leads to early peaking and decreased ability to reach their true potential. It takes a skilled coach to know when an athlete is ready to progress. For example, think about the differences between a child having difficulty because a skill is a new challenging motor pattern vs. the child who is having difficulty because they don't have the strength base to execute the particular skill. In the case of the first child, it is advantageous to continue attempts at practicing the skill. For the second child, continued practice, because of their lack of strength to execute the skill, likely will result in them developing a maladaptive movement pattern.

Seek out coaches who know, understand and regularly expose children to the fundamental athletic patterns in addition to sport specific training during their sport practices. Coaches who are working with children prior to the ages of 15 should be incorporating a good amount of athletic development into the majority of their practices. If your child only works on technical sport skill at their practices, they are missing the most important components of becoming a skilled athlete. The ideal sports program has an athletic development component built in. If you are unable to find a program that recognizes this as a priority, then it is best to seek out an additional athletic development program to augment their development.

Look for programs that are interested and willing to work with your son or daughter's goals and train him or her based on what their needs are, rather than what is in the best interest of the team or club. For instance, a young pitcher who has aspirations of elite competition has to manage the amount of pitching he or she does over periods of years. High volumes of pitching in younger years limits the health of their arm and can lead to serious overuse injuries. Coaches and programs should be well aware of this reality and should put the athlete's health and future goals before the team's needs. Furthermore, sports programs should always be willing to work with young children who are involved simultaneously with other sports. It is essential that the coach be willing to adjust volume and intensity of workouts to avoid overtraining. As your child nears mid to late adolescence, it then becomes important from a performance standpoint, for them to specialize and devote year-round training to one or two of their favorite sports. The adolescent that continues to enjoy many sports can continue if they choose to pursue a wide variety; however, at older stages, optimal performance in any particular sport will be sacrificed because of the lack of volume and focused attention on that particular sport.

As a parent, it is easy to get caught up in wanting your child to be performing at the highest level possible in the present; however, you must use restraint to not push your child too far. Again, the very act of pre-maturely accelerating your child is the very thing that will impede their ability to reach their full potential. With the guidance of a good coach, you let your child lead their own progression. If they are demonstrating the ability to consistently perform at any level, they are most likely ready to progress and be challenged at the next stage, regardless of "age groupings." In larger clubs or leagues, the child should be afforded the ability to "play up" or at least work on advancing skills with older groups. When there is only one level of talent or team, as the child demonstrates the need, the coach should provide him or her with more challenging skill sets. In the same regards, when a child is lagging behind on a team, the coach should be able to adjust for the individual by regressing the skills or movements.

Experts and scientists are for the most part on the same page when it comes to the development of athletes. All point to the importance of developing the athlete's skills during the times that they are most able to learn them, and the fact that talent is developed over the long term. The Canadian model, LTAD, is one systematic approach being used successfully not only in Canada, but in other countries as well. Despite the USA's lack of an organized athletic training system, there are programs and coaches out there who are slowly adopting the practices and framework of the Long Term Athletic Development Model. It is not necessary to find programs that adhere to the model itself, but it is advised to find programs and coaches whose training approaches are based on the development of your child's athleticism over the long term.

Utilizing the previous guidelines will give your child many advantages towards developing into a talented athlete. The information however is far from all-encompassing, I strongly urge parents to seek as much sound information and education as possible. For more information and resources please visit: www.VantageSportsPerformance.com

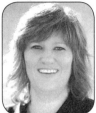

About Wendy

Wendy Breault is the Owner and founder of both Vantage Sports Performance and the Junior Olympic Volleyball Club, Minnesota Vantage Volleyball.

Wendy was a three-sport high school athlete and all-conference basketball player. She went on to play college basketball and earned a BA in psychology with a minor in exercise physiology. Wendy is trained in Functional Movement Screening and Corrective Exercise Technique by FMS. She is certified by International Youth Conditioning Association as a Youth Fitness Specialist and is a level 2 certified Youth Speed and Agility Specialist. She is currently in the process of finishing her High School Strength Coach Certification.

Although Wendy has coached multiple sports over a span of 20 years, her passion and interests have always been in the science and application of strength and conditioning, athletic development and in sports performance.

CHAPTER 9

Sports and Kids: Life Lessons Disguised as Fun

By September Woods

How often do you have an opportunity to do something with someone's "everything?" That's how a colleague of mine describes coaching children - and I think it's very true. Children are constantly developing mentally, physically and emotionally - as a coach for junior athletes, we impact their lives in a significant way every time we interact with them

Coaches are really in the mentoring business, not just the sports and fitness business. Although the focus is obviously on developing and improving the children's physical abilities, many side benefits come out of that process - important lifetime traits such as character, courage and confidence. The truth is that coaches change lives - and they also have a social responsibility to make a positive impact on the children entrusted to them.

At our Sports Performance Center in Barcelona, Spain, I've seen this principle in action every day. I see kids learning these life lessons in a way that's doesn't require lecturing about abstract morals. Instead, they absorb those lessons through normal physical fitness and sports activities - or, to put it simply, through *fun*. Because these lessons are learned in a positive and active way, they are retained throughout a lifetime. So, in this chapter, I'd like to share more about how kids learn from participating in athletics and sports development - and how the right coach can make a huge difference to the rest of their lives.

LEARNING THROUGH SPORTS

Our parents and teachers, of course, teach us valuable life lessons, but in a different way than how a coach does. I've always thought that learning through sports is a lot more practical. Kids are focused on real attainable goals and they put themselves to the test to achieve those goals.

It's said that children "learn through movement." Movement is a vital means of communication and expression, as well as learning; it helps children develop social, emotional and cognitive skills. And kids love to play sports. You know why? Because it is something they can get good at and succeed at. And with that success comes acceptance, praise, and recognition - the kind of positive feedback that every person wants and needs. When that happens, they dig in and try harder - resulting in sports giving them purpose, discipline and focus.

I know that from personal experience. I played many sports when I was a child; you name it, I loved to play it. Sports was always a huge part of my life - and I grew up to become a professional snowboarder. Those experiences definitely improved and changed my young life, it built my confidence. What happens in the gym or on the playing field ultimately gets played out in our daily lives as we grow older.

WHAT SPORTS TEACHES US

In addition to the values of respect, responsibility, teamwork and making a good effort, there are many life lessons that sports teaches our kids. Here are a few that I know I learned from my coaches along the way.

- **Discipline**
Sports requires that athletes set realistic, achievable goals - and develop the methods to achieve them. This results in a plan to win - and is a process that anyone can use in everyday life for any situation. Discipline is required to turn that plan into a reality. With discipline in place, you give your best effort and maximum performance. You don't let yourself off the hook when the going gets tough; instead, you keep pushing forward.

- **Dedication**
At our Sports Performance Center, we work on the basics with the children - agility, coordination, speed, change of direction, strength, etc. We focus on building athletes first - and then they can further specialize and become a basketball player, golfer, swimmer, etc. But, aside from the physical lessons, they also learn that they must fully dedicate themselves to the task at hand in order to succeed at it. Again, as they progress in life, knowing how to deliver that kind of dedicated effort will see them through many difficult situations, whether it's in school, work or their personal lives.

- **Teamwork**
Everyone has to recognize that they need to fulfill their individual duties to make the overall team a success - and that, when everyone does his job, they find success together. Teamwork means working together towards a common goal - which involves supporting one another, respecting each other's strengths, understanding their weaknesses, and losing your ego when the situation demands it. Humans are social creatures - and teamwork makes our lives easier and more rewarding.

- **Honesty**
If someone is slacking off and not giving a full effort, they quickly see that they're not only cheating themselves, but they're also cheating the entire team. Likewise, if someone is taking shortcuts and not being straight about how much they're actually practicing and training, they see that they're

shortchanging everyone who's counting on them to give their very best. There's no hiding the truth on the playing field - because coaches depend on their players to tell the truth and to live that truth in their actions.

- **Respect**
Win or lose, you will be held accountable and responsible for the decisions you made. That's why you must respect yourself first; then respect the game and its rules and traditions. People will respect *you* when you approach life in that way. That's how winners live their lives and achieve their dreams.

- **Humility**
Don't confuse being humble with not having confidence. They are very different things. When you're humble, you're open to new people, new experiences and new ways of thinking; you're not arrogantly dismissing the unknown because you're secretly afraid of it - *that's* a lack of confidence. The humble person is able to accept that another way may be better, another person may know something they don't, and an unexpected situation isn't something to run away from. Humility also allows us to take advantage of the wisdom of others as well as the advice and good sense of our family and friends.

- **Integrity**
Once you understand what is right and what is wrong, the next step is to have integrity and live your life with those values in place. Do the right thing regardless of the consequences. You may not know the answer to every question, or you may even make the wrong decision - but if you approach things from the right moral standpoint, you'll come out okay. You have to have courage to do the right thing even when no one is looking – and respond in a way that is honest and true.

- **Confidence**
If you don't believe in yourself, no one else will. Understanding and accepting your strengths and weaknesses allows you to be realistic about your abilities. Know what areas you excel

in, and don't be shy about contributing those talents for the greater good. The ultimate overall quality of any person's life is in direct proportion to their commitment to excellence. Confidence is required to make that kind of commitment.

WHAT'S WINNING ALL ABOUT?

Winning - and losing - builds character and teaches the most important life lessons. If you have a goal, you work harder. You learn to cooperate with others to reach that goal. When you have setbacks, you work at what went wrong so it doesn't happen again. You improve yourself. You learn sportsmanship. And you learn the importance of rules, the importance of playing by the rules.

When a child's parents or teachers lay down rules and restrictions, they often seem arbitrary and meaningless. You're in a classroom, so what's the big deal if you talk or chew gum or play on your cell phone? A kid can easily justify that kind of disruption - it's not affecting anyone else and the class is still going on as scheduled.

But, when you're playing a sport and you ignore a rule... well, bad things happen. You run out of bounds and suddenly there's a penalty. You commit a foul and a point doesn't count. If I tell you not to put your foot over a white line, if I told you why and we've practiced it a hundred times, and then you go ahead and do it anyway... well, you'll find out first-hand why you shouldn't have and not from me. The referee will quickly penalize your team - and that team will be wondering why you did something that you knew was wrong.

Breaking the rules could mean losing a game - there are immediate consequences for both you and your team. On the other hand, learning the rules and obeying them means you'll *gain* something - a better chance at a win and more respect from your teammates.

HOW PARENTS CAN HELP

Coaches are in partnership with parents who want to help their kids help themselves. I tell everyone, I can teach you how to do a push-up, but I can't do your push-ups *for* you. Parents naturally want the best for their children - they want them to be great at whatever they do and that includes excelling at sports. But until the age of about 18, kids are still developing - emotionally, and physically. You can't train a kid like he or she is a small adult. These are kids! Biologically and neurologically, they still have a ways to go.

Allow your child to find their passion for sports naturally. Don't push your sport onto them. It's important to let them make their own choices and find their own enthusiasms. That's what will drive them forward, not relentless hectoring and badgering.

Kids want to be active; they just need the inspiration, encouragement and the training. And the best thing about them is they never stop learning - so we never stop coaching. Sports has a lot to offer a child beyond fitness - the life lessons they learn through training and competing offers an incomparable preparation for their adult lives. So let your child do "something with their everything" - and they'll grow up to be great people as a result.

Isn't that what you want for your child?

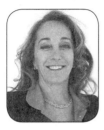

About September

September Woods is a native of Los Angeles, CA with 20 years experience in the sports and fitness business.

Currently operating a Sports Performance Center in Barcelona, Spain. First International Parisi Speed School Franchisee in Europe.

Current position;

General Manager of Parisi Speed School Barcelona, Sports Performance Center, and Golf Performance Center.

Specialties;

- Junior Coach
- General Physical Preparation Coach - all competitive athletes
- Individualized Metabolic Conditioning
- Athletic Based Strength Training
- Golf Specific Performance Programs
- Strength Training Program Design
- Total Body Conditioning

Certifications;

- Titleist Performance Institute (TPI)
- Certified Level 3 Golf Fitness Professional
- Certified Level 3 Junior Coach
- Certified Level 2 Biomechanics
- USA Weight Lifting (USAWL) Certified Sports Performance Coach
- Functional Movement Screen (FMS) Certified Exercise Professional
- Parisi Speed School Certified Performance Coach
- Power Plate Certified Fitness Professional Level 3

CHAPTER 10

The Right Fuel - The Right System

By Dr. Mark McCullough

The engines of some cars are built to run on premium - and when you consistently fill those vehicles up with regular, you're asking for trouble when it comes to that engine's performance. It won't burn lower-octane fuel as efficiently and over a long period of time, the engine itself can actually be damaged.

Well, human beings are created to take in a certain kind of fuel as well. Today's America, however, is dominated by artificial, processed foods that create problems for our own internal engines. That's what many of our children end up eating regularly - and that affects not only their fitness and athletic performance now, but their overall health for the rest of their life.

You may not be aware of just how much the wrong diet can negatively impact a child's life. If you want the best for your child both in athletic competitions as well as their adult lifestyle, this chapter should be a must-read for you.

MY OWN MISTAKES

Speaking for myself, I began concentrating my own energies in sports and fitness at the age of five. Unfortunately, I went about pursuing my physical health in exactly the *wrong* way.

I was a very competitive young boy and my parents encouraged this side of me. It all began, strangely enough, with the fact that I absolutely hated being in water when I was young. Even baths made my skin crawl. My parents were determined to help me conquer this phobia, so they put me in swimming classes - and that's where my athletic streak really surfaced. When I saw someone swimming fast, I immediately made it my goal to swim faster. Soon, I wasn't at all affected by my initial horror of H_20 – as a matter of fact, by the first grade, I was swimming competitively. During my elementary and middle school years, I also participated in baseball, football and basketball. As I was very coordinated for my age, I was pretty good at all of them.

Note that I said, "for my age." As I turned into a teenager, other kids began catching up to my skill level, which is a very common occurrence. But, along with being competitive, I'm also stubborn - so I drilled myself harder and harder to try and maintain my edge over them. It didn't work. All it did was burn me out physically as well as psychologically. High school was all about pain - because I ended up playing hurt in just about every game, as no one knew how to treat young athletes as they do today. Science and technology in that area had yet to fully evolve.

The experience, however, taught me that it's necessary to have the right mindset with specific goals, a plan with purpose, and a way to measure outcomes in the areas that will guarantee success. You need to know what you're doing and *why* you're doing it, instead of blindly battling on as I did.

And a large part of my ignorance back then was about how the kind of foods you eat affect your physical performance and health. I was always running with low blood sugar - which, in turn, caused me to always be hungry and always be eating. That's because I was eating too many carbs - causing my system to burn sugar instead of fat. My "engine" didn't work efficiently as it does now. If I had started out with the right foods, my body would have been more efficient and reached the higher level of fitness that it's at now.

THE NUTRITION CRISIS

Beyond burning fat efficiently, the right nutrition will help your children escape other more serious health problems late in life. No doubt you've heard about the rising rate of obesity in our society, as well as the alarming rise of cases of Type 2 Diabetes. A bad diet can also bring on strokes, heart attacks and numerous other life-threatening critical diseases and conditions.

There is also the growing body of evidence that indicates Twinkies just might be as addictive as cocaine and nicotine. It sounds crazy, but, according to Nora Volkow, director of the National Institute on Drug Abuse, "The data is so overwhelming the field has yet to accept it. We are finding tremendous overlap between drugs in the brain and food in the brain." Twenty-eight scientific studies and papers on food addiction were published in 2011 alone, according to a National Library of Medicine database.

What happens is that highly processed, mostly artificial junk foods that contain empty calories cause a neural feedback loop in a person's brain that closely resembles the neural feedback loop of a person on drugs. Not only that, but junk food junkies continued to crave the stuff long after they've eaten it. And the more junk food that is consumed, the more the brain builds up a tolerance for the food - which means even more junk food is needed to produce the same effect on the brain. Sound familiar?

That's why it's good, even, crucial, to avoid training children's brains at an early age to respond in this incredibly unhealthy manner to incredibly unhealthy food. I'll get into more specifics about diet in a little bit - but first, let's take a "big picture" over-view of the 'what's crucial to our human health.'

AVOIDING DISCONNECTS:
YOUR CHILD'S WELL-BEING

To begin with, the human body is controlled and coordinated by the brain and the spinal cord, which constitutes the central nervous system. In order for your heart to beat, your lungs to breathe, or even for food to digest, your three-pound brain is required to have an excellent relationship with every one of your tissues and cells - in order to allow optimum health and efficiency. If a disconnect develops between the brain and the corresponding seventy-five trillion cells in your body, the result is dysfunction instead of function, disease instead of ease, and degeneration instead of regeneration.

How does that kind of disconnect develop? Well, there are actually any number of ways it can happen, but, for simplicity's sake, I'm going to talk about three big causes: *trauma, toxins*, and *thought*.

Trauma, believe it or not, can begin as early as birth. No matter if it's a vaginal or caesarian birth, both are considered a "medical intervention." During these procedures, a significant amount of pulling to the neck can cause damage to that part of the body, as well as to the spinal cord of the child. And, because it takes months for the child to creep, crawl, or walk, that neck ends up healing in the wrong way, creating nerve blockage and nerve system interference. This particular disconnect makes the system work a lot harder; it also affects the soft tissue of the spinal cord, nerves, and organs as well as creating uneven wear and tear on the bones, discs, and corresponding joints.

If the spinal cord is not assessed at an early age, a child's system can become less and less efficient - and imbalances in the musculoskeletal system may be created. These imbalances can materialize in the form of unforeseen damage that disguises itself as overuse injuries. On the other hand, when the spine and skeletal system is checked and treated, optimal, full-leveraged function can be obtained.

Toxins can come in the form of anything that can penetrate your system and affect your biochemistry in a destructive manner. I call this "chemical interference." What you put on your skin, what you breathe, and what you ingest are all examples of chemical interference. And for athletes who want to achieve the highest levels of health and fitness, the most important way that interference can happen is through eating the wrong foods.

To me, the most important cause of disconnect is **thought**. Every child, through the use of their minds, employs the tools of listening, touching, feeling and experiencing; through those tools, they create mental patterns and interpretations that they will engage in for the rest of their lives. That fact should make coaches, trainers, and yes, parents, all very aware that they have an integral part of shaping the future of kids in either a positive or negative way.

In my practice, I've discovered that children love direction, accountability, and boundaries - as long as they know the reason why for each of them. You don't have to give complex college-level explanations for everything, but just provide simple nuggets of information that they can easily process and truly understand. Between doctoring, coaching, and consulting, I have advised many kids to success and let the parents do what they do best....love their children.

The important thing for parents to realize is that children make lifestyle choices primarily by modeling their parents' behavior, not through instruction by them. If what you do directly contradicts what you tell your child to do, this sends out mixed messages which challenges the basic logic they have at that young age - and that causes them to question. That's why I always say, "Rules without relationship lead to rebellion."

For example, how parents eat connects directly to how their children eat. If you're telling them to eat fresh fruit when you're snacking on donuts, again, they'll be confused and they'll jump for those Krispy Kremes when you're not looking. The whole key is to give the kids proper food choices, and help them understand, as well as take ownership of, how those foods provide positive outcomes for their daily lives.

FOOD 101

Here's a little primer on what I consider to be the necessities of a proper diet.

• Water

As you remember, I had regarded water as one of my arch-enemies at the age of five. I now regard it as one of my body's best friend. Water is one of the most important "foods" imaginable; proper digestion, nutrient absorption and elimination are all dependent on drinking enough of it on a daily basis. It also lubricates and cushions joints, ensures healthy skin, helps remove toxins from your body as well as helps control your body's temperature.

But you have to drink enough of it. Believe it or not, if you're peeing yellow, you are dehydrated. The basic rule of thumb is this: Divide your body weight in half and drink that many ounces per day. For example, if you weigh 200 pounds, you should consume 100 ounces of water every 24 hours.

Other beverages I recommend drinking, besides distilled, fresh spring or filtered water, are almond milk, fresh fruit and vegetable juices, organic herbal teas, organic herbal coffee and coconut milk.

• Carbohydrates

Carbs are designed to break down slowly into simple sugars and provide us with the energy we need to do what we have to do during the day. There are good carb foods and bad carb foods - and they can make the difference between how efficiently your system burns fat.

Foods containing good carbs include:

- Fruits - Apples, bananas, berries, etc.
- All natural whole grains
- Vegetables such as peas and squash
- Potatoes and sweet potatoes
- Foods containing bad carbs include:

- Corn (most is genetically engineered, which creates inflammation)
- Refined or processed sugar
- White breads
- Corn starches
- White flour
- Soy

• Proteins

Proteins are on the opposite side of the food family of carbs. They're the most abundant source of amino acids and are needed for muscle, organs and nerves. Almost all of our tissues are made up of proteins - so proteins help us build, heal and repair those tissues. As with the carbs, there are protein foods that are good - and bad - for us.

Foods containing good proteins include:

- Organic eggs (from free-range chickens)
- Organic free range chickens
- Organic grass-fed beef
- Turkey (free-range)
- Fish (wild caught)

Foods containing bad proteins include:

- Pork - pigs eat everything including car tires
- Shellfish (bottom dwellers - they eat muck ...yuck)
- Non-organic beef, eggs or fish (omega 6:3 fatty acid ratio imbalance which creates inflammation)
- Caged chickens (inflammation☹)

• Fats

Fats are used for cell membranes, balancing hormone production, and transporting essential vitamins. Fats also reduce your overall hunger level - causing you to eat slower and less.

Foods containing good fats include:

- Nuts such as almonds, brazil nuts, walnuts and pine nuts
- Fish oils
- Olives
- Pumpkin seeds, sesame seeds and sunflower seeds
- Avocados

Foods containing bad fats include:

- Homogenized and pasteurized milk and cream
- Vegetable oils
- Shortening
- Table salt (not a fat but an ingredient in most fatty foods)
- Fried foods
- Trans fats (genetically engineered to increase shelf-life, not your life)
- Artificial flavors, preservatives and most artificial sweeteners (toxic ingredients associated with fatty foods)
- So how do you practically apply the above information? Well, here's a suggested blueprint for your daily diet that will enable you to gain the energy you need for you daily activities and create a healthy and efficient system for burning fat instead of sugar:

  - **Morning:** Eat foods with high to moderate carbohydrates, low in proteins and low in fats.

  - **Afternoon:** Transition to foods with low carbohydrates, low in proteins and low in fats.

  - **Evening:** Go for foods with zero to low carbs, moderate to high protein and moderate fats.

- Finally, I'd like to add a few more thoughts about the importance of vegetables in a child's diet (as well as an adult's!). Vitamins and minerals are necessary for virtually all reactions to occur in the body. And there is no better way to consume these than by eating vegetables that are all colors of the rainbow (but, preferably, green and leafy). This food group not only gives you an incredible amount of fiber but also great amounts of water, vitamins, minerals, and antioxidants, all of which are required to sustain life. Vitamins and minerals do not supply energy; they are both, however, required in energy metabolism in the body.

That means that, when vitamin deficiencies are present, body functions are reduced and health is impaired. That's why kids, coaches and parents need to be schooled on the importance of this vital food group. And, no, supplements do *not* replace the consumption of these life-giving foods. Whole food has a nutrient communion between the actual food and body. And when it is consumed, the body recognizes it as fuel to be ingested and converted from fuel to usefulness.

That's not to say that supplements are not important, though. But supplements should only be prescribed by a healthcare professional that has thoroughly evaluated the child's lifestyle factors such as food consumption and physical activity and is targeting specific vitamin and mineral deficiencies.

In the beginning, man and woman were provided here on Planet Earth with bountiful amounts of fresh, nutritious foods to eat and clean water to drink. As our technology improved, we began to travel down a slippery slope to where we now fill ourselves with fast food, processed foods, frozen dinners, artificial sweeteners and diet sodas. Big industrial farms crank out meat with antibiotics and hormones, and claim that it's all safe.

We need to take a step back from what's the most convenient and available in today's supermarkets - and take a closer look at the kind of diet that creates a healthy child who lives a quality life long after the "big game" of their senior year is over and forgotten.

If you'd like more information or have a specific question about

how your child can achieve optimum health and quality of life, I invite you to contact me at:
nextlevelmichigan.com and
ivaluelife.com

Let's be as careful with how we fuel our kids as we are with how we fuel our cars.

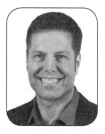

About Dr. Mark

Dr. Mark McCullough is a Michigan native who earned his B.S. degree in Chemistry in 1991 and began his career as a bio-analytical scientist. After 5 years of Research and Development, Dr. McCullough went back to school to pursue his doctorate degree.

A graduate of Palmer College of Chiropractic in 1999, Dr. McCullough established his clinic and within the first few years of practice, become one of the largest Chiropractic clinics in the state of Michigan and operates one of the largest Natural Health Clinics in North America. In addition, he is a nutritional consultant as well as being a certified specialist in both Youth Fitness and Youth Nutrition by the International Youth Conditioning Association. Dr. Mark is also pursuing a Master's Degree in Herbology.

Dr. Mark is a contributor to the *New York Times, USA Today*, and *Wall-Street Journal* Best-seller *One Minute Wellness*. Dr. McCullough co-founded Next Level Health, a program to help doctors start up and run successful "patient-centered" care to their respective communities. Dr. Mark is founder and CEO of both Pure Health Solutions, LLC, a nutritional consultancy, as well as a Crossfit Affiliate in Battle Creek.

Dr. Mark also served as the Team Doctor for the 2005 IBL Champion - Dr Mark McCullough Family Chiropractic Battle Creek Michigan Knights from 2005-09 and is currently the Team Physician for Team Active Cycling and Multisport Team as well as the Priority Health Cycling and Multisport Team. Dr. Mark's mission is in serving his patients and helping potential students of Natural Whole Body Health realize and achieve their potential as Doctors.

His innovative strategies, inspiration, and passion for helping people are the foundation to his thriving practice in Battle Creek, Michigan, as well as the many clinics he consults with around the nation. His passionate work began when his own son was diagnosed with autism. And through a customized plan involving numerous lifestyle-enhancing strategies, his son is now a mainstream teenager excelling in music and will be attending Hillsong College in Sydney, Australia in 2012.

Dr. McCullough has hosted weekly radio shows for years. His incredible contributions to his local community of Battle Creek that he serves has allowed him to be invited as a guest speaker to many of the schools that teach Health Care around the country. At seminars, conferences, and media appearances throughout North America, he shows people how to apply his Whole Body Wellness Solutions that will get you to the Next Level in health, happiness, and life.

In addition to being a devoted to husband to Missy and devoted father to Jake and Macy, Dr. Mark is an outstanding athlete. He was sponsored by a type-1 diabetic team, Triabetes, in 2009 and was not only an Arizona Ironman Finisher, but has been slated as one of the fastest diabetics to do ironman distance triathlon in the world. Other endeavors include the 2009 Huff 50K, 2011 Run Woodstock 50K, 2008 and 2009 Steelhead 70.3. Dr. Mark placed 4th and 3rd in the 2008 and 2009 Bayshore Half Marathon, and has achieved National qualifying times in Master's swimming in both 2009 and 2010.

CHAPTER 11

Building Better Athletes

By Carlo Alvarez

Athletes want to be successful, they want to win and at times are willing to do whatever is necessary to make that a reality. We've seen the stories, watched the news and stared at the images of athletes holding the championship trophies, celebrating the culmination of all the hard work they've put forth for that moment. The moment they become a champion. These moments of ultimate success on the field come from the dedication, hard work, commitment and discipline of an athlete, team, school and community, to do what is necessary to work together and accomplish great things.

The title of this chapter, *Building Better Athletes*, is a simple statement of what you'll find here: insightful ideas to help you build championship caliber athletes through better strength and conditioning programs. These ideas can assure you a more structured program as you work towards your own championship.

MY JOURNEY BEGINS WITH A VIDEO

Over the last 18 years, I have been blessed to be able to work with athletes at the high school, college and professional level. It has been an extraordinary journey, and it all started as I watched a highlight video in the University of Cincinnati weight room. As part of our freshman curriculum in Sports Medicine, we were introduced to Coach Mickey Marotti and his training philosophy. He started the class by showing us a video of the basketball team going through grueling strength and conditioning workouts. He explained his training philosophy and what it took for the Bearcat athletes to represent the school on the court. He talked about being mentally tough, disciplined, hard working and committed. I was sold. The next day, I went to my advisor and changed my major. That's how my story begins. A motivational video changed my whole perspective and track in life.

I spent three years as a student assistant at the University of Cincinnati. After college, I was hired at the University Of Notre Dame where I worked with all 26-varsity men and women's sports. I left Notre Dame and went to work with the Cleveland Indians, responsible for developing player training plans and coordinating Latin American athletic development programs and internships. In 2002, I was hired as the Cincinnati Reds head strength and conditioning coordinator, responsible for the major league, minor league and Latin American operations. In 2005, I became the head strength and conditioning coach at St. Xavier High School, where we have developed what is considered one of the top high school strength and conditioning programs in the country.

Having the opportunity to work at every level of sports, has given me a unique perspective in how we should train our young athletes. My intention with this chapter is to provide you insight into our football-training model. A model that has developed conference, regional, state and national champions, as well as dozens of all-conference, district and state 'first team' players. All the success we have achieved on and off the field is due to an organized plan that is carried out diligently by everyone in our school and community.

GAME PLAN

The purpose of this chapter is to help administrators and coaches develop long-term athletic development programs. I will discuss concepts that will help you structure an annual training plan with more confidence and allow you to create programming that will help you improve the performance of your athletes. Everyone has different challenges as they look to improve their strength and conditioning program from year to year. My goal is to provide a basic off-season strategy that is simple to follow and can be adjusted based on your specific needs.

As Director of Strength and Conditioning at St. Xavier High School, all of our off-season strength and conditioning planning is based on four simple goals: building team unity, reducing the likelihood of injury, enhancing performance and increasing work capacity. Before we can determine what our teams off-season needs are on any given year, we always take into consideration some basic tenets that provide the foundation for our strength and conditioning programming.

We understand that the development of a yearly strength and conditioning program has become an important component in our success as a high school football program. Due to our demanding schedule, it's critical that we have our team well conditioned year-round. A comprehensive annual strength and conditioning plan has become a necessity in our program. As you look at the top programs in the country, high school or college level, the successful programs have usually followed a structured yearly training plan. The yearly training plan usually includes components such as: flexibility, mobility, strength, speed development, agility, conditioning and nutrition education.

As you begin to outline your off-season strategy, consider your specific organizational challenges, program structure, and implementation system prior to determining your annual plan. I have found that organizing, structuring and systemizing our off-season program is like building a brand. We start by defining our philosophy and expectations; is the program physiologically and psychologically sound? We establish our expectations, to help our athletes become better in all facets of athletic development. We define how we want to be perceived by our competition and build on our skills and strengths to provide our unique type of football player. There are no secrets here. We want to be perceived as a team that is disciplined, strong, fast, agile, smart and tough; a team that strives for the highest level of personal development and athletic achievement, while consistently competing for championships. What's your brand?

IMPLEMENTATION MODEL

Establishing a "power base" is critical in setting your program in the right direction. All efforts should be coordinated and organized intelligently for a definite purpose. We like to use the Flywheel Concept as the basis for our implementation model. Imagine a huge flywheel as you apply great force to rotate it. At first it doesn't move, but through great perseverance you get it to move, if only for an inch. You continue to apply force until it reaches a satisfactory speed. As you continue to apply force, the wheel builds momentum and can sustain itself with little push.

We like to think of strength and conditioning as the hub of a wheel, with the administration, head coach, sports medicine, nutritionist, staff, athletes and parents as the spokes on the wheel. To make the wheel move all spokes have to be moving in the same direction. Getting everyone on the same page takes patience and perseverance, but is well worth the process. We focus on making sure everyone on the wheel is on the same page, pushing in the same direction, with the same goals and objectives. We focus on education, motivation and constant updating of our accomplishments. People involved in the process want to know how our athletes are doing and what's it going to take to get to the next level. It becomes a support system, which works together to support mutual goals. The interaction and educational process allows us to build a strong community and fosters a sense of ownership from everyone at the school.

ANNUAL PLAN

What separates a good athlete from a great one? We ask ourselves this question often and have come to realize that it comes down to four basic components: psychological makeup, physical ability, sound mechanics and comprehensive conditioning. You can develop these four components through an annual training plan, which can maximize the performance of your athletes by dividing the training year into manageable segments.

You can breakdown the annual training plan into four major phases: post-season, off-season, pre-season and in-season. Each phase has specific goals and objectives that lay the foundation for the next 'more intense' phase. Exercises and drills will have to be organized into a yearly, monthly, weekly and daily basis to peak players as they go into the season. When designing programs for young athletes, your goals should be to develop the athlete's function and versatility, improve motor abilities, coordination and balance, and improve overall physical development. The level of competition, size, strength and speed at the high school level has increased exponentially over the last decade. To keep up, today's athletes must work year-round to improve the skills necessary to compete. I'll provide a basic breakdown of the post-season, off-season and pre-season phases; it's goals and objectives, to help you build your annual training plan.

POST-SEASON

The post-season phase is a critical period in the overall annual training plan. It's the first stage in the annual training plan and begins the day after your last game. Your main focus in this phase should be on the total evaluation of the program. Before you can start developing your off-season plan and training your athletes, you have to evaluate what you accomplished during the prior season. The purpose of evaluating is to understand the impact of your program, how to improve implementation efficiency, and be able to produce comparisons between programs.

The evaluation process should begin with a thorough assessment of your injury reports, training and rehab protocols, reconditioning and execution plans and successful implementation of the overall program. Meet with your athletic training staff and review the season injury reports to determine areas of concern. This will allow you the opportunity to determine specific strategies to eliminate or at least be proactive in diminishing these types of injuries in the future. You always want to start your off-season training program with your players as injury-free as possible. You might not have 100% of your players ready on day one, but it will give you a good sense of where you stand as a unit and what is being done to get everyone injury-free and on the same page. Make sure that you determine what players need immediate surgery, rehabilitation, or individual pre-habilitation protocols prior to beginning your first day of training.

The next step in the evaluation process should be to assess the overall impact of your training program. Every coach needs to be honest as to what they want to accomplish with the strength and conditioning program. Do you want your athletes to be injury-free, bigger, faster or stronger? You should hold end-of-season meetings to determine goals and identify specific needs of your program. The meetings will provide a foundation as you move into your off-season training phase.

OFF-SEASON

The second stage of the annual plan is the off-season development phase. Depending on how far your team made it into the playoffs, this phase can last anywhere from 20-30 weeks. Over a six month period, you can complete anywhere from 60 to 120 workouts with your football team. The objectives of this phase are to determine player strength and limitations, and enhance the team's level of flexibility, mobility, strength, power, conditioning, speed and agility. Determine what is most important, and build your foundation focusing on those specific needs through player assessments and performance testing.

Every training program should begin with assessment and testing of athletes participating in the program. Coaches might misconstrue the purpose of testing by believing the results obtained are a measure of how successful they will be in the future, instead of merely representing a means of checking various components which contribute to the success of the team – components which athletes should try to improve through a comprehensive athletic development program. What test you decide to use should be reliable and objective. The testing will help you establish the teams' initial performance levels and determine where you need to focus, as you begin your training program.

Once you have completed your testing, evaluate the data and establish individual goals with your athletes. It's much easier to achieve success as a team when everyone understands what each individual must accomplish. Keep the goals realistic, progressive and challenging. You can continue to monitor their progress through an annual testing cycle

PRE-SEASON

The pre-season is the third stage of the annual plan and will focus on sports-specific training. Being organized during this phase is important and must be monitored on a daily basis, as you might have to make constant adjustments. Focus on improving team communication channels and getting everyone on the same page. From a training perspective, volume will drop progressively, allowing for an elevation of training intensity. The volume of work for strength development is reduced and the training, conditioning, speed, agility and plyometrics become more sports and energy specific. You must focus on improving and perfecting technique and tactical elements that will be emphasized during double sessions in the early part of August. All exercises included in your weekly menu must be of high quality and have a maximum training effect. Exercises should facilitate a general transfer of movement patterns for the individual to have a maximum training effect.

During the pre-season phase, the total volume of fundamental work on the practice field must be monitored to accommodate total volume of work during the strength and conditioning scheduled times. This is the time of year where you need to be smart about not compounding volume, intensity and muscle breakdown just for the sake of adding more work. Smart training protocols, nutrition, and recovery strategies become critical in reducing injury and lost time.

Start to build a monitoring system for injuries that might occur during this period. Your relationship with the medical and athletic training staff becomes critical. Daily injury reports allow for individual training plans. This allows everyone on the team to be on the same page. Being pro-active with how you deal with injuries eliminates any athlete from falling through the cracks, and prolongs a reconditioning that can have the player on the field sooner rather than later. We like to make sure that injured body parts don't affect our overall training program. Having daily injury reports allows us to progress injured areas accordingly, and still develop gains throughout the body. Injured body parts do not mean an injured body.

Raise the intensity during the pre-season phase; increase your conditioning, speed, agility and plyometric work, while maintaining consistency with your strength training. Maximize downtime to work on recovery strategies and monitor total practice volume to adjust your own programming.

FINISHER

Developing an off-season strength and conditioning strategy can help you build momentum as you prepare your players for the upcoming season. Focus on your specific organizational challenges, program structure, and implementation system. Work on continually educating your teams and athletes on the importance of building upon the training phases in the annual plan. Break the year down into small segments, which allows the players to see incremental improvements in every stage of their training. Take into consideration the athletes' age, pace of individual development, the demands of the sports and level of physical fitness. A well-rounded program should implement a safe, competitive and educational training atmosphere to allow the young athlete to improve. Make sure you motivate through education and goal setting, as you make an impact on the athletic performance of your team on the road to the championship.

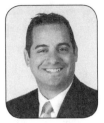

About Carlo

Carlo Alvarez, is regarded as one of the top strength and conditioning coaches in the country, specializing in performance enhancement training for athletes at the high school, college and pro-level.

He began his coaching career at his alma mater, University of Cincinnati as a student assistant. During his studies at the University of Cincinnati, Carlo became strength and conditioning coach at St. Xavier High School, where he implemented innovative and successful programs. In 1998, Carlo ventured to South Bend, Indiana to the University of Notre Dame where he evaluated, designed and implemented programs for male and female varsity athletes. He left the University of Notre Dame to become Assistant Strength and Conditioning Coordinator for the Cleveland Indians where he was responsible for developing player training plans and coordinating Latin American athletic development programs and internships. In 2002, Alvarez became Head Strength and Conditioning Coordinator for the Cincinnati Reds, responsible for the major league, minor league and Latin American operations. During his time with the Reds, he developed one of the most comprehensive and recognized athletic development programs in Major League Baseball and Latin America. In 2005, Alvarez became the Head Strength and Conditioning Coach at St. Xavier High School, where he has developed what is considered the top high school strength and conditioning program in the country. Since 2005, St. Xavier has won two Ohio Division I State Championships, three Regional Championships and a share of the National Title.

Carlo is the founder of Ethos Athletics and consults with companies and institutions including Nike, Gatorade, Vizual Edge, EAS, PR Soccer Elite, Humana, HIMA Health and Wellington Orthopedic, helping them with testing, product and program development. He serves on the advisory boards of the University of Cincinnati College of Education and Health Services, Cincinnati State Health and Information Technology Department and HIMA Health, as well as is a contributing writer for Total Health Breakthroughs and Fitness Editor of The Healing Prescription.

CHAPTER 12

Technical Training, Techniques and Their Application

By Christian Isquierdo

There are very few resources for the un-athletic player. There are scarce resources for the child that is plunged into the competitive, cut-throat chase of the early status seeking parents and clubs that take the best athletes, throw a ball in the middle of field and reward the biggest, fastest, strongest most aggressive player when he or she kicks it into the back of the net.

At LeftFoot Coaching Academy, a private soccer training school, I've developed a recipe for success that integrates technical movement training, coaching strategies that support the techniques and brought everything into successful applications for my clients on the field. This philosophy was designed to develop athleticism and integrate correctional exercise within a supportive coaching environment. Combined with a foundation of mental discipline, we created a path for hundreds of local soccer players to go from the lowest teams to the top level of play. These players experienced what I now refer to as the Foundation Series of LeftFoot Coaching Academy's model of Great Player Development.

Maia Lundstrom was a gawky, uncoordinated, aloof player that was cut from the lowest of five U11 teams. She couldn't strike a ball, dribble, run or squat to save her life. From a Functional Movement Screen perspective, she would have been a 0. She was passed from clinic to clinic, club to club, until her father was introduced to me in the winter of 2007. Maia was cut from the local super-club team because she couldn't play in the field, and so her father sought me out with the intention that she would never be cut again from a team because she couldn't play in the field as a goalie.

Maia and I created a three-pronged strategy to get her onto the top team as a field player:

1. She was going to be creative with the ball.
2. She was going to be a deadly ball striking machine and
3. We were going to make her so technically sound in multi-directional speed techniques that she would have the foundation of skill to build on as she grew into her body since she was only 12.

Three years later, Maia earned several accolades on her way to becoming one of the elite goalkeepers in the state at a leading soccer academy. She now plays half the time in goal and the other half in the field.

Another player, Gabriel Bland, was the daughter of an English soccer player who was born premature. At the time of our intro-duction, Gabby couldn't accelerate, stand on one leg or execute a single leg lunge. Her footwork, shot and speed were less than appealing. I cut Gabby from my second team while at the local super club during the first years of beginning LeftFoot Coach-ing Academy.

My first team had the best athletic soccer players at U12. My second team had average players that still needed work. Gabby didn't make either team. When her mom asked me why, I gave her seven technical skills that I wanted to see in players on the top team. Her mom stated that this was the first time ever that a coach had given specific, technical feedback to her about her daughter, and so we started a coaching relationship that was geared toward getting Gabby onto that team, even though I knew it would take years. This started a private coaching strategy that was bent on replicating the success that I had with Maia and transitioning the success to Gabby, while still integrating soccer skills with athletic development.

Most coaches would take these players and start them touching a ball, dribbling and gaining a touch, or they would teach them a series of moves and ask the players to perform them. And that's what I used to do prior to meeting Maia.

Now, almost 200 players and five years later, I have created what I now refer to as the Foundation Series of the Great Player Model of Development.

The Foundation Series is a six-step process that involves the idea of working backwards from what Great Players do.

At LeftFoot Coaching Academy, I outline several significant characteristics of Great Soccer Players.

Great Soccer Players are:

1. Creative with the ball.

2. Great in the air.

3. Accurate and full of power while striking the ball.

4. Fast in Body and Mind.

5. Balanced in task and ego-oriented goals.

6. Aware of Vision and Movement in multiple directions on and off the ball.

7. Passionate and Effective communicators.

Great Players can do all of these things well at the highest level. And while we break down the tasks into the techniques and the measured skills of how we teach our players to be great, we start with a Foundation of Skills that every player must learn and master. Our success comes from these Foundational Skills in combination with the Values of our company (which help players go from the last team to first team), and how other coaches can create successful experiences for players of every sport.

The Foundation Series starts with multi-directional speed, or what's commonly referred to as Lateral Deceleration, within the principles of movement in the International Youth Conditioning Association literature.

When I first began teaching Lateral Deceleration to Maia I noticed that all of the ball skills she had brought into her soccer skills didn't correlate with how the body moves. As a Martial Artist, form leads to application, yet in the soccer world we often just use what works. Maia could not hold a static Lateral Deceleration stance in a stationary sequence without falling, and so by spending countless hours progressing her technical understanding of the sequence of steps within a static application of Lateral Deceleration, we began to integrate "stances" into the application of ball skills and ball striking at the Academy.

In most soccer books and courses, technique is messy and has very little sequencing that flows across platforms. While some pioneers are trying to pin down names of "moves," the study of the actual movement of the body is often left out of the discussion of the technique. By integrating the IYCA principles of movement and multi-directional speed to evaluate many common soccer "moves" – how they are taught by so-called experts, actually damages the youth player over time.

Using the Lateral Deceleration technique at the Academy, we combine static and dynamic movement of the lateral deceleration stance of the body with the common move called the step-over, through a series of progressions we refer to as a five-step learning sequence – called the Step-Over Sequence.

I combined these moves so that I could teach form and application at the same time – using a ball to create an integrated experience. Unlike using ladders to teach rhythm and balance, we use the step-over sequence to teach comfort with the ball, acceleration, deceleration and game application all at once. We also integrate both the left and right feet in stopping and restarting a moving ball. Cutting and changing pace in a repeated sequence on both sides dynamically with a ball is a process I refer to as "looping", where the same movement is executed without pause and for an extended period of time. The trainer can include changes in duration, intensity, and rhythm.

The Step-Over Sequence includes seven dynamic progressions with the ball: Static replication of the technique with a dead ball, Dynamic repetition of the technique in short bursts of speed with a dead ball, Dynamic repetition with a moving ball, Dynamic looping with a moving ball, and then Rhythmic movement with a moving ball. Players finish the sequence with applications against partners, and then integrate into game application.

THE FOUNDATION SERIES #1:
LATERAL DECELERATION

Learning and applying the Lateral Deceleration stance on and off the ball is the first step for students at LeftFoot Coaching Academy to master. It creates the foundation of all of our movements with and without the ball, as well as creates a series of sequenced progressions that students can adapt to new skills. From this stance we can then add more technical skills.

THE FOUNDATION SERIES #2:
QUICK-SIX TOUCH

The second process in the Foundation Series is called Quick-Six Touch, and we use our Hesitation Sequence to teach it. That way, each student progresses their understanding of Linear Deceleration techniques into a series designed to create six different surface touches of the foot with linear movement – while touching the ball and changing rhythm.

Our Quick-Six Touch theory suggests that ball skills for soccer players are not the combination of a library of moves, but are really the application of over twelve different surfaces of the foot touching the ball at speed, rhythm and deception. There are also six different types of touch that, when combined with different surfaces, create a flurry of skills and combinations for players. How we introduce the Quick-Six Touch is by using a second sequence of skills which overlaps and combines skills into faster movements.

The Hesitation Sequence entails a series of five "moves" that when combined, create over ten different surfaces and five types of touch. What coaches can do is take the concept of "overlay" and "looping" and progress those with foundational skills of their own sport.

THE FOUNDATION SERIES #3:
LOW-INSTEP DRIVE

The third step in our Foundation Series is what we refer to as the Low-Instep Drive. A driven ball in soccer is produced by striking the ball dead center with a locked ankle. The ball will travel with no spin on a single straight line just below knee height for ten to forty yards. For most youth players this is almost impossible. Which is why it is third in our series because it takes the longest to teach, but it creates a foundation for the next three progressions.

The Low-Instep drive includes several dynamic movement sequences that most athletes lack: jumping, landing, extension, pelvic tilt, ankle mobility, the ability to decelerate on a single leg, balance and then connect both the arm and leg in a sudden thrust of contra-lateral expansion and contraction. We also have issues associated with the hips and rotational movements with 90% of our new students.

Both Gabby and Maia had no rotational movement of either their hips or their upper body. Gabby had a slight hunch in her upper back and her leg lacked any mobility in both the ankle and knee extension. She swung her leg straight through the motion from a linear approach and her arms were dangling by her side. At the point of teaching Gabby, I had just nailed down a series of nine steps that progressed the application of striking the ball. At that point, I was starting to replicate an execution of techniques of allowing the student to practice the Low-Instep Drive.

Using a series of progressions and exercises to expand on each topic within the form, I was able to begin replicating the success I had with Maia for Gabby. I began to modify corrective exercise movements into the technique of the Low-Instep Drive.

For instance, Gabby would stand on her left leg and then extend her left hand over her head while at the same time flexing the knee back to touch her right buttocks. At that point she would bring her knee through to touch her chest while her left arm would cross her body, all while keeping her back straight. This exercise would be given a series of sets and reps, and done before and after striking a stationary ball. It would also be done while moving in a "looping" linear fashion, but then also combined with lateral movement. I would expand and make it harder as I continued to work with her by combining movements on the ball and the angles of approach.

Gabby and I continued to work together, but expanded our work at the same time that I was coaching my team of players. While I was building a super team, I was coaching a group of players from another team within the same age group, league and community. I started teaching them the same things I was teaching my teams and finalized the last three concepts of the Foundation Series.

THE FOUNDATION SERIES #4:
FIRST TOUCH SPATIAL AWARENESS

A player's ability to see space and allow their first touch to capitalize on attacking that space is critical to understanding tactical development. Unfortunately the current way that soccer is taught is not how soccer is played!

Most coaches still teach players to trap or stop the ball without understanding that the youth game requires a speed of play that is consistent with full court pressure basketball. While the professionals can stop the ball and look to assess the game, youth players with unlimited substitutions need to have different technical and tactical skills.

The first touch and spatial awareness of the player is a critical skill that has to be taught and constantly applied to tactical situations. Even from a bio-mechanical stance, several techniques that are popular in clubs are too slow and predictable to help players deal with the fast-paced dynamic nature of the game. By applying and integrating lateral directional movements associated with cross-over steps and the directional step in lateral movement, the first touch development is critical in developing creative players.

THE FOUNDATION SERIES #5:
AERIAL CONTROL

Players are brainwashed these days to "keep the ball on the ground" or "settle the ball first" with a preconceived notion that soccer is only played on the ground. Often players feel that "control" is only at the bottom of their foot and they have an awkward feeling when the ball is in the air.

Unfortunately, a majority of problems that occur in the game have the ball in the air! Being able to control the ball in the air with multiple surfaces and in a variety of directions is essential for players that want to play at the highest levels. Strikers who can dribble the ball but can't head or volley the ball are basically worthless. How many times have you seen players shank the ball as it comes out of the air, or miss hit a header? It's because we have outdated ideas of the game and outdated methodologies. By integrating correctional movements with the ball, players have shown an increased comfort not only "in" their body, but also with the ball moving in the air.

THE FOUNDATION SERIES #6:
MEASURING SUCCESS

Most players have grown up with the American parent's view of soccer success: Boot it, chase it, pass it, get it and destroy the play! Our players then learn to measure their success based on the impact they have on the game as it relates to how they can boot the ball, chase down attackers and run fast. While at the top levels of the game the measures of success are far more intricate; players and families can't find ways to set reasonable goals within the game without tracking things like "moves" or "goals" and wins. At LeftFoot we teach players the fundamentals of the game at the highest levels and encourage players to see success on the field in different ways.

Finally, while we've created a series and philosophy within Left-Foot Coaching Academy of how we want to teach and develop players … it is ultimately about how the player responds to technical training. The Foundation Series is nothing if game play and application are not integrated with the total experience of technique. I've found that the player's experience with the game and all of its movements and opportunities is never fully integrated unless the coach or the game is keeping technical skills and application front and center.

Games of all sorts with and without the balls are critical to finding movement opportunities and repetitions high. At LeftFoot Coaching Academy, we try to emphasize that all sessions include at least 100 technical applications of movement each session. Touches on the ball exceed or reach toward 2,000 and strikes on the ball exceed or reach 500 strikes. Our goals and our opportunities to reach our targets have to be measured and increase opportunities for players to get better each day they come to us. Without technical application, we've done nothing for the future of the player – and our players could not go from last to first.

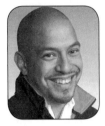

About Christian

Name: Christian Isquierdo, M.A.
City: Minneapolis, Minnesota
Company: LeftFoot Coaching Academy
Website: www.LeftFootCoaching.com
Work Phone: 612.545.5273

List Education, Honors and Awards:
IYCA, Youth Fitness Specialist, 2010
IYCA, Youth Speed & Agility Specialist, 2010
Master Class Series, Player Psychology & the Modern Coach 2008
USSF National "B" 2008
USSF National "C" 2007
USSF National "Y" 2005
USSF National "Y" Instructor Certified 2005
USSF National "D" 2005
NSCAA National Diploma 2004
Master of Arts, Naropa University
Bachelor of Arts, New Mexico State University
Class AA Girls Varsity HS State Champions 2010 #1 Nationally Ranked team
MYSA Summer State Champions 2010
Grand Prize Winner of Coca-Cola Live Positively Campaign 2010
Section 6A Assistant Coach of the Year 2007
Class A Boys Varsity HS State Champions 2006

Christian's passion is not just for the best a player can be, but the great player within every student. As a student of the game and a passionate ambassador, Christian takes every player through a personalized session and tries to integrate life lessons, movement, the unknown splendor of the universe and the amazing qualities of the ball with what it means to be a great player.

With a number of accomplishments on and off the field, Christian's favorite accomplishment has been creating a "soccer home" for every level of player in November 2010, when he and 24 families opened the first 10,000 sq ft. soccer specific training facility - dedicated exclusively to students of the game to play year-round in Minneapolis, MN. Over 60 players finished their first year at the Academy being promoted to the next level team.

CHAPTER 13

Getting to the Next Level

By Paul Rozzelle

You hear it all the time in sports, "I want to get to the next level." Now for some people, this could mean simply advancing up to the next step in the progression of sports, going from high school to college, college to pros, Junior Varsity to Varsity, etc. Or for others, it is going from bench player to starter, starter to All-District or All-District to All-State. Each one is obviously different from the other, but they however, have one underlying common assumption, and that is that the athlete must elevate their game or athletic ability to new heights. Owning my own sports performance facility, I encounter this daily and work towards assuring that all the athletes in our facility will reach new heights, regardless of what level on which they begin. We have athletes of all ages, sizes and genders. Some are the area's best and most talented, while others have to work extremely hard to improve limited ability. Regardless, each person has and will always have, a "Next Level" that they can reach.

An example of this is of one of my past top athletes we had in the facility. He was a local standout high school football player – who actually had committed to the University of Utah before even stepping foot in our facility. So right away, we already knew we had a dynamic talent in front of us. He came to us because he wanted to be better than what he already was. He was a Safety who had a decent first step along with strength, and ran in the mid 4.6's when he started with us in the forty. We had him for four months before he was supposed to report to Utah to begin his college career. After talking with him, it became obvious what his goals were. He wanted to improve his speed (both linear and multi-directional), improve his footwork, and improve his strength (not only in performance but for his recently reconstructed ACL which he tore in a previous season). From a coaching standpoint, we knew if he put in the hard work and effort, all of his goals would be met. We laid out a plan of action and he followed it to perfection. Four months later, this young man was lifting numbers he never lifted before, getting times he had never gotten before on footwork and speed drills, and his knee never felt better. Oh I almost forgot, he dropped his Forty time to the low 4.5's and actually hit 4.48 at one point before he left for school. Fast forward another couple months, and he is one of the strongest and fastest of his positions amongst the other players his grade as a Redshirt Freshman, and has a definite opportunity to see significant playing time in only his second year based solely on his athletic ability and as the position coach put it, "Excellent Footwork!" With the great strength staff at the University of Utah, he would have easily been ready to reach his goals after a full year in their outstanding program, but he took the opportunity to set goals early and work towards them before he left for school and put himself into position to stand out early for his coaches, and will soon see the fruits of his labor. He made it to his next level.

Not all athletes that walk through our door are elite level athletes however. Actually, those are extremely rare. The question is, what do we do with the kid who is slow, has zero coordination and limited strength? That is where we, as coaches, earn our paycheck. And truthfully, these are the ones I get the most enjoyment out of. Now that we talked about our elite athlete above, let me tell you about guys on the opposite end of the spectrum. I got a phone call from the dad of a freshman high school athlete who had heard about our program and wanted his kid to participate. He tells me his son plays football and that is all he wants to do, but during the conversation he keeps bringing up the point of his sons lack of footwork and lack of speed. So we set up a time for him to come in for his first session, and let's just say ...this young man struggled. He struggled with basic footwork drills, had almost zero speed and pretty much everything we did that day seemed to prove extremely difficult. Now, with that being said, I did notice something about this young man through all of this, HE TRIED AS HARD AS HE COULD IN EVERY-THING! Even when he was tired, he would give the best he had. After the workout we talked for a little while about what he wanted to accomplish and it was interesting to hear his response. He said, "I just want to be better."

Here we have a kid with the worst feet this side of the Mississippi, no speed and he didn't say anything about improving footwork or speed, he just wanted to be better. So where the elite athlete presented to me exactly what he wanted to improve, the below-average athlete had no clue where to begin. So as a coach, it was up to me to map out his goals and his progression plan of what we had to do, in order for him to get "better." That athlete got completely immersed in our program. He was training three times a week for a better part of the year until football camp rolled back around. He made small steps and progressions every month and what we saw was cumulative growth in his athletic performance. He never made huge strides or did anything that was eye opening. Just one day, we started to notice fluid movements. We started to notice the steady improvements in our Movement Rating Evaluation and his footwork actually started to be a strong suit. Before we knew it, we had a starting Junior Varsity Linebacker on our hands.

Now what I haven't told you about this young man is that I am friends with one of his coaches. When he first got involved with our program, I asked this coach what he thought about him and what he could work on. This coach looked me in the eye and said, "Great kid, but good luck. He's one you can't help." A year later, my assistant and I are now the Speed Coaches for this young man's high school football team as well as working with the Men's Baseball team, and Women's Softball team. This is strictly because of the turnaround in this young man.

In both cases, each athlete progressed to their individual next level. One was preparing himself to play at the highest level of College Football and the other was trying to see more playing time on his Junior Varsity team. Although the end results were different, the process remained the same. Set goals and work diligently every session to improve towards those goals. The focus was placed purely on the process as opposed to the outcome.

So how do we establish a way to do this with every athlete? Each athlete that has committed to our program has become a faster, stronger and overall better athlete. So how is this done day-in and day-out regardless of who walks in our door? Well, we developed our own system to insure that each and every athlete will reach their "Next Level." Now before you read further, there is no "magic bullet." These 5 steps are things you have to work at. They are things you have to create and things you have to provide to each and every one of your athletes EVERY DAY!! Each coach should take these five things and make them daily practice – and if done correctly – you will see optimal results from every athlete.

1. GOAL SETTING

We have all heard of this one before. But we have heard it because it is still the most important. Nothing great is accomplished without the intent of accomplishing greatness. What we did with the above athletes was establish where they were, and where they wanted to be. We established a known point and started moving forward from there. When an athlete is not quite sure where to start, we have to start asking them questions. What does that mean? What needs to be better? How do we make it better? Once the athlete starts to think like this, they start to understand the concept. Instead of saying, "I want to be a better athlete," have them say "I need to improve footwork, coordination, and overall functional strength." From here we can begin to now make sure that their program meets each of the individual smaller goals and gives them clear direction as to what they are focusing on in each and every workout or practice.

2. ACCESS PROGRESS

Our facility does this with our own Athlete Movement Rating that Brent Johnson, my fantastic Assistant Coach, and I created. Brent was and still is one of the best athletes I have ever seen or worked with, as he was an All-American Wide Receiver during his college days. We perform a six-event assessment that measures the athletic ability of each of our kids every month. And it assigns a rating to each athlete so they can see where they are themselves compared to previous months, as well as compare themselves against kids their own age. Now for other coaches, this "Assessment Tool" may be different. We focus on movement and speed as our niche, so we developed something that evaluates that specific thing. We have seen fantastic results from this, and it provides motivation for each athlete and provides immediate feedback for their hard work. It also provides information to us as coaches that either confirms the effectiveness of our program or if we have to change certain things in our programming to achieve the goals we set out for our athletes. Every coach should have something that the kids themselves can see, something tangible, on their improvements.

3. CREATE A CULTURE

As a college strength coach, I have always said creating an environment and culture of hard work, dedication, and achieving success was extremely easy at the college level.

When working with a college team, competition is built in. In college, everyone is talented. An athlete has to do one thing to get motivated to practice and work hard and that is, look around the room at the other players and realize, "Wow. If I want to play, I have to step it up." At lower levels, this can be a little harder as the sense of urgency is not necessarily present with younger athletes. But we, as coaches, can absolutely help with this. We can set up reward systems that encourage strong performance. We can promote healthy competition between athletes that show it's ok to want to win and be the best. You are never going force that "light switch" to go off in an athlete by telling them they have to work hard. As a former athlete, I heard that stuff since I was 6 years old and I didn't really understand what that truly meant until I had my "light switch" moment. It didn't happen from a speech or some coach yelling it at me. It happened on my own time. So as coaches, we have to create an environment that will create that moment for each athlete. And each kid is different, they will reach it on their own time so we have to make sure that every single day we are creating the culture that will promote this moment, not force it.

4. COMMUNICATION

Open dialogue is a must. After our monthly assessments we talk to our athletes. Are they happy with their progress? What do they need to do better? Do they feel the training is worth it? We have to coach these kids, but they need to be able to talk to us. If something is off with their scores, we have to find the cause of the problem. We cannot just blindly berate them for the lack of performance. When an athlete feels like they can speak with you honestly, they are more apt to give you everything they can, because they know you truly care about them not only as an athlete, but as a young person as well.

5. GIVE IT YOUR ALL EVERY DAY

YOU HAVE TO BRING IT!! Day-in and day-out, you have to be the best coach you possibly can be. As I am writing this, I just worked with over 50 athletes in one day. This included my college baseball team and then the kids I have that come to our facility ages 6-18. These are back-to-back training sessions for six straight hours. No breaks, just a coach in the trenches trying to make athletes better. I know that there are coaches reading this that understand the exact feeling that every coach will get from time to time. You're a little tired (ok, you are exhausted), and maybe you killed the first 5 sessions with high intensity and passion. But if you don't show up for the last session you have failed as a coach, as a leader and as a mentor. You have to be everything to everyone ALL THE TIME!! Not part of the time. Athletes will notice the slightest difference in your demeanor. Scratch that, KIDS notice. Your job is to be the professional they look up to that is guiding them on this journey. Kids are the ones that are going to be up and down. There is no room for the coach to be as well. Bring it every day!!

If you can truly follow these 5 steps everyday, it will absolutely help your kids and athletes achieve success that they have never achieved before. I can tell you this because we do it every day. Some days are harder than others, but these steps drive us every time we stand in front of a group of young men and women and we see results. We are not promising professional contracts or college scholarships, but we can look parents and kids in the eye and say we will make you better than you are right now, and then once initial goals are met, we re-evaluate them and move on to the next goal. ...The "Next Level."

The Next Level is not some mythical place that only a certain few reach. It is a real, tangible place that if guided correctly, every athlete can reach. Again, no matter if it's the kid who doesn't play on Junior Varsity or the kid who wants to compete for Collegiate National Championships, it is about the process.

If the process is performed correctly, the next level is just a commitment away.

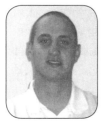

About Paul

Paul had a vision for providing a sports performance and fitness facility 10 years ago as an athlete in high school and had a vision to provide elite level training to people that normally do not have access to it whether it be financial or geographical. Paul was an active athlete throughout high school being a part of 2 State Championship Golf Teams as well as playing American Legion baseball. Paul went on to Appalachian State University where he graduated with a Bachelor Degree in Business Administration with a major in Health Care Management. Paul also participated in both Mountaineer Club Baseball and Golf while at Appalachian State. Paul is a certified Speed and Agility Specialist, Youth Fitness Specialist and Youth Nutrition Specialist.

Paul currently is Strength and Conditioning Coach for Catawba Valley Community College Baseball. He also served as an Assistant Coach there in the program's inaugural year where the team reached a national ranking of 14th in the program's first year. Paul also is the Speed Coach at Bandy's High School working with the Football, Baseball and Softball teams. Paul has worked with elite athletes of all levels from Division II to the Professional ranks.

Paul, alongside Brent Johnson created the Athlete movement rating, which is utilized in their facility to help grade and access athletes on movement performance. Both coaches are currently working towards bringing this outstanding evaluation tool to facilities and coaches around the world.

Paul also serves as the Director of Sports Performance at the Dynamic Fitness and Performance center, which he helped co-found in 2011. This is an all-inclusive facility that not only caters to athletes of all levels, but adults and children as well. Paul also serves as the Head Coach for Athletic Revolution Hickory, which is the youth fitness and performance model that the DFPC uses for kids ages 6-18.

Paul is also a devoted member of the International Youth Conditioning Association, which is the worldwide leader in youth fitness and athletic performance. The IYCA validates research and provides appropriate examples of practical application for working with young athletes and youth participants at large. The goal of the IYCA is to establish industry norms with respect to safe, effective and clinically sound means of optimally developing injury-free, emotionally sound and functionally gifted young athletes and participants.

For more information, please visit the following websites:
www.dynamicfitnessnc.com and
www.athleticrevolutionhickory.com

CHAPTER 14

Speed Training Warm-Ups
How to warm-up the body and Central Nervous System for sprinting activities, and why both are important for good performance.

By Eric K Dixon, USATF/IAAF Sprints

I believe the warm-up should take about 20 - 30 minutes to raise the core temperature and get your muscles ready for sprinting. The warm-ups are done from low intensity to high intensity with each segment and rep. The intensity of the workout scheduled for the day will determine what dynamic warm-up drills I will do. Also, if I continue to do the same drills over and over, I will get bored with them and my body will adapt and there's no growth for the Central Nervous System (CNS). The CNS is also a critical component that needs to be warmed up, and is usually forgotten about – not just in the warm-ups, but in the entire workout/practice (another article). For the most part, I stick with a 4.2.2 or later in the season a 6.3.3 followed by the dynamic warm-up drills at least #1 through #6 (see below). For myself and the athletes I coach, I do not promote static stretching until after you've completed the whole warm-up routine. I'm not against static stretching; I just don't like it done when the muscles are cold. I believe static stretching places microscopic tears in the muscle fibers, which can cause serious problems later. I explain this concept to my athletes with the rubber band vs.

muscle analogy by taking a rubber band out of the refrigerator and stretching it. What happens to the rubber band? Could it break or tear? Think about it (of course, I could go into more detail on this topic but that's not for today). In addition, you're stretching the muscles in ways that you're not going to use it. Even a hurdler will not have his or her leg fully extended when going over hurdles. Their knee is slightly bent. Also, you increase the chances of diminishing your power output with static stretching. Again, the rubber band analogy; if you pull and hold it too long, it will eventually decrease in its power output and not travel as far when released. This is because you've stretched out the elasticity (Stretch Shorting Cycle or SSCs). I feel that static stretching does have its place. However, it should be performed only if necessary and after your "Warm-up routine" or after the workout. Now, if you're a hurdler, high jumper, etc… or need the extra stretching because you're just genetically very tight, it's ok to do static stretching but again after your warm-up runs and dynamic warm-up drills …and only in moderation.

THE NERVOUS SYSTEM

The Nervous Systems consist of two parts, the Central Nervous System (CNS) and the Peripheral Nervous System (PNS). However, to keep it simple we will just focus on the combined function of the CNS, i.e., Neuro-muscular system (NS) – Neuro = Nerves and Muscular = Muscles. A whole different subject, though related, is the theory of specificity or motor learning. FYI: There is no generality of abilities. Each sport has its own distinctive set of movements and patterns. Therefore, the warm-ups for sprinting activity should be geared to take advantage of these movements and the body's, i.e., muscular as well as the neuro should be warmed up accordingly. Again, the problem is that this area is vastly overlooked in the warm-ups and sometimes even in the training program.

The CNS acts as a two-way highway. It sends signals from the brain to the muscles and from the muscles back to the brain. One of the things I teach my athletes is to listen to your muscles.

Yes your muscles talk to you; you have to learn to listen to them. This two-way highway helps coordinate your movements, regulate your force production, rate of speed, balance, control, etc… The CNS is the highway and the impulses your brain sends and receives to and from the muscles are the cars on the highway. Let's say 50% = 50mph, 75% = 75mph, and 100% = 100mhp. You get the idea? If your cars are traveling at 50% then you're setting the governor/traffic of the highway at 50mph.

I see a lot of coaches do slow Dynamic Warm-up drills to get the kids ready for sprinting activities. Sorry coach, all Dynamic Warm-ups are not created equally. There are slow Dynamic Warm-ups and fast Dynamic Warm-ups. If you want to get ready for sprinting activity, you need to do the fast ones. You're not just warming up the body but the highway that's using it. Again, if you're warming up the body at 50% of its top speed then you are setting the governor at 50-55%. Thus, you're setting the athlete up for injury or a subpar practice session when they try to go all out. Think about it, you're warming up the body slowly but you're going to sprint with it. You are not preparing the body properly for the planned activity. You need to warm up the muscles in the way they will be used in the practice session of your sport, event, or race.

In addition, if you continue to use the slow warm-ups drills, you're also telling the brain to send the signals to the muscles at a slower pace. This is also counterproductive to preparing the body to go faster in the future. Furthermore, if you consistently train at 60%, your top speed will be about 65%. The athletes will not reach their full potential in top speed because they are training at a lower speed. Of course, there are other factors like proper form, force productions, etc… again, material for another article. Now, I'm not saying you need to train at 100% all the time, because that will burn out the athlete and will also cause injuries physically and mentally. This is where you need to plan your training seasons – yearly, monthly, weekly and daily sessions. This process is called "Periodization." It should predict when you should train hard (85-95%), when to train medium (75-85%) and light days (60-75%). This will all depend on what type of training you are working on and when i.e. Extensive tempo, Intensive tempo, Power Speed, Event Running, Speed, Speed endurance, Strength endurance, Special endurance 1 & 2, and Endurance. Note: all the endurances are different aspects of endurance – they are not the same! These workouts are also contingent on the Energy systems being trained, i.e., Aerobic, Anaerobic, Alactic, Glycolytic and Lactic acid tolerance... and all will have an effect on the athlete's neuromuscular system.

Now back to the car and highway analogy. When you are doing your warm-ups, you also teaching the neuromuscular system where the off-ramp is for that particular muscle. Some people have problems with coordination and balance because the brain is trying to find the right off-ramp faster than it has been trained to react... Remember, you trained it to go slow. However, when performing the warm-ups drills at a faster pace, you're teaching the brain where to send the signal and how fast to send it – with the proper reaction time to perform the drills correctly. This translates directly into the technical skill and speed of motor learning. And yes, it is imperative that the drills be performed correctly! I've seen a lot of athletes doing them wrong. Remember, you're warming up the neural pathways for proper sprinting mechanics. If the athletes are doing them incorrectly, then they are teaching the brain to send the signal down the wrong path/off-ramp. Or you're teaching it to send the signals in the wrong sequence. Thus, bad form and sprinting mechanics equal slow performance, balance and control. Please remember you are warming up the whole body.

Yes, it is a lot of work, but remember you could have a potential Olympian in your group. So you need to do your homework and get it right the first time.

THE WARM-UP ROUTINE

The "Warm-up routine" serves several purposes:

1. **Warm-up:** To get the blood flowing and warming up the muscles in the way they're going to be used for the upcoming sprinting session.

2. **Communion/Mental Prep:** This is where you get ready mentally, physically and the CNS for what's to come – "Speed work."

   a. Getting inside your head (psyched up): it's up to you what works to get into pre-launch mode!

   b. Preparing your body (warming-up): you need to get the fuel systems flowing and engine revving!

   c. Systems check (CNS): you need to get the communication lines open from brain to muscles. "Mission Control, we are a 'go' for launch!"

3. **Talking inventory:** As you start off slowly and are increasing speed with each rep, you're taking an inventory of your system/body. As the blood starts to flow through parts of the body that may not have had much stimulus during the day, you may start to feel twinges and soreness from the last few workouts. That's your body telling you that something's not quite right (good or bad). It's up to you to decide if you should keep going or shut it down! Be smart – listen to your body. It knows more than you!!! What you have to decide is if it's a good pain or bad pain. Conversely, what you don't want to do is ignore it and start compensating for the precondition or restriction. Doing so will lead you down the path of more problems and/or injuries later. As athletes, we will automatically compensate and ignore it. Don't do this! We should Identify with it and know it's there. Remember, you only have two choices: a). Keep going with no compensation to your form, or b). Shut it down!

4. Form work: You're also teaching your body the proper form when you're going slowly as well as fast.

WARM-UP RUNS

4.2.2 or **6.3.3.** All done on the 100m straightaway

(4.2.2) =

4 x 100m – *(Continuous jog easy)* working on form/arms: elbows at 90-degree angle (between upper and lower arm) on your sides and not coming across the body.

Jog 100m, turnaround, jog back 4 times at about 50-60% of your top speed.

Walk 100m.

2 x 100m – *(Continuous jog faster pace)* working on form/arms faster.

Jog 100m, turnaround, jog back 2 times at about 60-70% of your top speed.

Walk 100m.

2 x 100m – *(Buildups)* working on form/arms faster.

Sprint 1st 100m at 70-75% of your top speed, then walk back 100m.

Sprint 2nd 100m at 75-80% of your top speed, then walk back 100m.

If a 3rd is required, i.e., 6.3.3 then sprint 80-90% of your top speed then walk back 100m.

Note:

If you're running faster than 75% of your top speed (for most of you), you should be on the **balls** of your feet with toes up **(dorsal flex)**. You're sprinting and should get into the proper sprinter's form and slightly leaning forward. If you're running less than 70% of your top speed, then you are not on the balls of your feet; you're jogging.

DYNAMIC WARM-UP DRILLS

1. Distance is about 25m–40m depending on the season and your conditioning.

2. Do two reps of each at the beginning of the season, increasing to 3 at the end of the season.

3. Once you have the form down correctly for the drill:

    a. First rep should be 60-70% of your top speed.

    b. Second rep should be 70-80% of your top speed.

    c. Third rep should be 80-90% of your top speed.

4. Example: Ankleling for 30m

    a. 1st at 60-70% of your top speed.

    b. Walk back 30m.

    c. Repeat 2nd at 70-80% of your top speed.

    d. Walk back 30m.

    e. Repeat 3rd if necessary at 80-90% of your top speed.

    f. Walk back 30m for next drill.

BASIC DRILLS

1. Ankleling
2. A-Skips
3. High knees
4. B-Skips (cycling)
5. High Knee Butt kicks
6. Straight Leg Bounds
   a For Speed
   b. For Distance
7. Fast Leg Skip (single leg) right leg up, left leg back)/walking or running
   a. One step cycle

    b. Two steps cycle

    c. Three steps cycle

8. C-Skips

9. High knee carryovers

WHY 4.2.2 OR 6.3.3?

A lot of athletes and coaches ask me: "Why the 4.2.2 as opposed to a long continuous jog for a warm-up? " I believe anyone who's preparing for an explosives/sprinting type workout should warm up the body in the way it's going to be used. The CNS/Neuro-muscular system needs to be close to full stimuli/impulse to truly benefit from the workout. If not, you're just going through the motions; your body can be sluggish, or worse, you risk injuries. In addition, you should do a 4.2.2 because most of us (sprinters) have very short attention spans. I know I really have to con-centrate harder on my form if I'm continuously jogging 2 laps or more. By the end of the first 200m, our form is gone and we are just jogging and not thinking about what we are doing. The problem is we are teaching our body this is what it should do when it's going 50, 60 - 70% of our top speed. When fatigue sets in during your sport/event/race, guess what your body's going to do form-wise? What you've been teaching it! In most cases this **type of training** is not very efficient for sprinting, and will have a negative effect on your times. Think about it: a 4.2.2 = 1200m warm-up.

Note:

Sprinters should not do long distance jogs for warm-ups. That's "old school" and reason for another article.

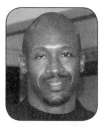

About Eric

Coach Eric Dixon has competed and coached Track, Speed and Agility for over 30 years, concentrating mainly on sprinting events (60m-800m). In recent years, his educational focus has been on Sport Specific Speed Training and Sports/Strength Conditioning Training. He's trained youths and adults in Baseball, Football, Soccer, Gymnastic (vaults and floor), Tennis, Volleyball, Skeleton, Cross Country and Track.

Eric Dixon is CEO and head coach of Tachyon Track Club and Tachyon Training Center. Coach Dixon has held the assistant coach positions at the High School and Collegiate levels. In his last 5 years of coaching, he has coached several nationally ranked youth athletes; American Masters record holders, and World Masters record holders. Coach Dixon has coached one athlete to a number 2 National Youth ranking in the 110 hurdles and coached the Orange County, CA high school (sophomore) female 200m record holder and qualifier in the 100m and 200m for the US Area Youth Olympic Selection Trials, Arlington, Texas – April 2010. He has also coached both the 2010 and 2011 Orange County Championships 100m winners.

Coach Dixon also coaches the Athena track team: a National Masters Women's Track club which currently holds five World and American records in the 4 x 200m, 4 x 400m and 4 x 800m relays. He also coached one Masters Sprinter (W71) to American and World Indoor/Outdoor records in the 60m, 100m and 200m.

Coach Dixon competes for USA Track and Field in the Master's Men's Division sprints (60m to 400m) in National and International competition. A Sports Strength Condition Trainer, USA Track & Field (USATF) Level 2 Sprints/Hurdles, Relays Coach and USATF/IAAF (Youth Specialization) Level 2 Coach. He is also one of 26 coaches in the US accepted into the IAAF Level 5 Coaches Academy (Elite Coach) Program for Sprints and Hurdles. He is certified to coach Elite Youth and Adult athletes for International level competition via USA Track & Field and the International Association of Athletics Federations (IAAF). In addition, he is a spokesperson for the *USA Track & Fields Win With Integrity Program* and director of *USA Track & Fields Coaches Education Programs: Level 1 Schools* for the Southern California area (where we coach the coaches).

For additional training articles, Warm-ups video clips, Speed training video clips, Weight training video clips or updates to this article, please contact: Coach Dixon or go to: www.TachyonTC.net.

Got Speed,

Eric K Dixon
USATRACK&FIELD Level II Sprints/Hurdles/Relays Coach
USATRACK&FIELD Level II Youth Specialization Coach
RCS Speed/Agility Trainer & Sports/Strength Conditioning Trainer

C: 949-636-9234

E: TachyonTC@cox.net

W: www.TachyonTC.net

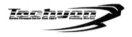

CHAPTER 15

Off-Season Strength and Conditioning for High School Football

By Richard Bell

There is a ton of information that exists regarding how to physically prepare football players for the grind of the game. Throughout my 16 years of coaching, I have always believed that it is not always about the X's and O's of a great program that is the sole contributor for one's success, but the coaches' ability to combine the science, their experience and intuition – that makes a program really go.

In the winter of 2011, I was finishing up a session with an athlete, when I was approached by a very concerned parent who wanted to know if I could work with her 17-year-old son Jonathan, who would be entering his senior year of high school Football that fall. Mrs. Harris calmly explained that despite numerous letters from major Universities, Jonathan's on-field performance in 2010 was well below his expectations.

I quickly scheduled a face-to-face meeting involving both parents and Jonathan, so we could put together an off-season football schedule that would not only have Jonathan crushing the competition on the field, but wowing the recruiters in the stands as well.

When I finally got the opportunity to meet Jonathan, I was quickly amazed at how tall he stood, 6'4"and with hands that would make a softball vanish if he held one. During our meeting I asked Jonathan to answer the following questions:

Questions:

1. What have you done in the past?

2. Why didn't work?

3. What are you willing to do differently this time?

Answers:

1. Lots of bodybuilding-type programs to add more size to my frame

2. Because even though I did add size to my frame, I became a much slower football player at my positions. (Linebacker and Left guard). I was dominated by opponents smaller and faster than myself, and my performance really suffered during the two-minute drills in close games.

3. This time I want to get the proper coaching and instruction that will allow me to be quicker and more explosive to the ball and opponents.

At the conclusion of our meeting we agreed that Jonathan would meet with me 3-4 times a week for the next 15 weeks – beginning with three days of physical testing. Jonathan had already set a goal to be in top physical shape for his visit to the University of Miami football camp coming up in June.

THE FOLLOWING TESTS WERE PERFORMED ON THREE SEPARATE DAYS

Day 1

Assessment Drills Performed: Lower Body

1. Stick overhead squat – To assess stiffness and range of motion in the hip, ankle and thoracic spine

2. Supine Faber – To assess stiffness of the muscles in the groin area

3. Supine Knee Flexion – To assess stiffness of the hip in flexion

4. Single leg squat – assess hip stability and gluteus maximus and medius strength

Assessment Drills Performed: Upper body

1. Seated thoracic Spine Rotation Range of Motion – To assess thoracic spine rotation left to right

2. Supine shoulder internal Rotation Range of Motion – To assess shoulder internal rotation range of motion

3. Supine shoulder external rotation – To assess shoulder external rotation range of motion

4. Standing scapula upward rotation – To assess scapular upward rotation, which is influenced by serratus anterior strength.

Day 2

1. Height: 6'4'"

2. Weight: 205lb

3. Body Composition: 22.8%

4. Power Clean: (1rm) 185lb

5. Box squat (1rm) 250lb

6. Bench Press (1rm) 200lb

Day 3

1. Vertical Jump: 25'
2. Med Ball Overhead Toss: 20'
3. Standing Med Ball Chest Launch: 18'
4. T-test: 9.5 sec
5. 5-10-5: 5.8 sec
6. 300-yard shuttle: N/A

Note: Due to fatigue, Jonathan was not able to finish the 300-yard shuttle run.

PROGRAM DESIGN

Phase 1: Accumulation Program

Days per Week: 4

Length: 4 weeks

Introduction:

Football players love to train in the weight room, and this is great, but my ultimate goal through this journey is to make sure that Jonathan's newly developed size, strength and power will be functional. An accumulation phase is defined as a higher volume of workload aimed at basic abilities such as endurance, strength, and general patterns of movement technique (which depends on the sport – Issurin, 2008). Like all programs, each phase will build off the other, leading to what should be a bigger, stronger and faster football player.

The following program is designed for two upper body lifts per week and two lower body lifts per week.

MON	TUE	WED	THUR	FRI
Foam Rolling	Foam rolling	Off	Foam rolling	Foam rolling
Mobility work	Mobility work	Off	Mobility work	Mobility work
Lower body lifting	Upper body lifting	Off	Lower Body lifting	Upper body lifting
Conditioning work		Off	Conditioning work	

Monday

Foam Roll lower body

1. Quadriceps
2. Hamstrings
3. TFL
4. Calf's

Mobility Drills

1. Ankle Mobs 2x5
2. Squat to stand 2x5
3. High knee walk forward lunge 2x5
4. Kneeling rock backs 2x10

Exercise	Sets	Reps	Rest
A1 Low cable split squat	3-4	8-12	90
A2 Single leg RDL	3-4	8-10	90
B1 Db Step Up off-set grip	3-4	8-12	90
B2 Reverse Back Extension	3-4	8-10	90
C1 Db Reverse Lunge	3	8-10	75
C2 Low cable rope pull through	3	8-10	75

Conditioning Session:

D1. Sled backwards dragging	4	50 yards	100
D2. Sand Bag Carry	4	50 yards	100

Tuesday

Foam Roll upper body

1. Thoracic Extension 2x10
2. Lumbar Extension 2x10
3. Lats 2x10

Mobility Drills

1. Side lying thoracic extension 2x10
2. Side lying rotation extension 2x10
3. T-push up with extension 2x5
4. Scapula wall slides 2x10

Exercise	Sets	Reps	Rest
A1 Fat bar incline press **(3' grip)**	3-4	8-10	100
A2 Band assisted Chin Up **(Heavy Band)**	3-4	8-10	100
B1 Standing cable 1-arm press **(Staggered foot stance)**	3-4	10-12	90
B2 Seated face pulls	3-4	10-12	90
B3 Band pull apart – I put this in as a form of active recovery in between sets.			
C1 Bent over trap-3 lift	3	8-12	75
C2 Farmer walks	3	40 yards	75

Wednesday

Soft tissue work 30-45 minutes
After school

Thursday

Foam Roll lower body

1. Quadriceps 2x10
2. Hamstrings 2x10
3. TFL 2x10
4. Calfs 2x10

Mobility Drills

1. Ankle Mobs 2x10
2. Squat to stand with overhead extension 2x10
3. Elastic band Side step 2x10
4. Wall Hip flexor mobilization 2x10

Exercise	Sets	Reps	Rest
A1 Trap Bar Deadlift (Off 4'podium)	3-4	8-10	90
A2 Glute-ham-raise	3-4	8-10	90
B1 Barbell step up	3-4	8-10	90
B1 Swiss ball triple Threat (supine)	3-4	8-10	90

Conditioning session:

C1 Sled dragging	4	50 yards	100
C2 Kettlebell Overhead carry	4	50 yards	100

Friday

Foam Roll upper body	Mobility Drills
1. Thoracic Extension 2x10	1. Side lying thoracic extension 2x10
2. Lumbar Extension 2x10	2. Side lying rotation extension 2x10
3. Lats 2x10	3. T-push up with extension 2x5
	4. Scapula wall slides 2x10

Exercise	Sets	Reps	Rest
A1 Overhead log press	3-4	8-10	100
A2 Db Farmer walk	3-4	40 yards	100
B1 1-arm standing Db Press (neutral grip)	3-4	8-10	90
B2 1-arm bent over Row	3-4	8-10	90
C1 60 degree Incline Db Superman	3	8-10	75
C2 Side lying Db External Rotation	3	8-10	75

Notes: At the conclusion of this Accumulation cycle, Jonathan reported having much better work capacity and had put on 3 ½ pounds of muscle. His body fat had dropped to 19.6% as well.

PHASE 2: INTENSIFICATION PROGRAM

Days per Week: 4

Length: 3 weeks

An intensification phase is focused on developing specific abilities – usually with a reduction in volume and an increase in intensity. An intensification phase would focus on those specific exercises that more closely resemble your sport. Goal for the next three weeks will be to move heavy loads in an explosive manner. This will teach the nervous system how to recruit the "high threshold motor units," which are responsible for fast twitch muscle fiber recruitment.

Because the body adapts very quickly to a given rep range, frequent variation in repetition prescriptions is necessary to ensure optimal progression. The following is the repetition prescription we used during Jonathan's phase 2 Intensification cycle.

Workouts: 1-2: 4-5 sets x 6-8 reps (focus is more on lower body)

Workouts: 3-4: 4 sets x 5-7 reps (focus is on upper and lower body)

Workouts: 5-6: 5 Sets x 4-6 reps (focus on upper body core lifts)

Note: Day 5 was an un-loading day and day 6 was used to re-test Jonathan's weight room lifts to determine his new 1rm in the core lifts.

Monday

Foam rolling lower body:
1. Quadriceps
2. Hamstrings
3. TFL
4. Calf's

Mobility Drills:
1. Ankle Mobs 2x5
2. Squat to stand 2x5
3. High knee walk forward lunge 2x5
4. Kneeling rock backs 2x10

Exercise	Sets	Reps	Rest
A. Cambered bar box Squat	5	6-8	120
B1 Reverse Lunges off 4" block	4	6-8	100
B2 Single leg reverse Back extension	4	6-8 each leg	100
C1 Db Russian step up	2	8 each leg	90
C2 Swiss Ball hip Extension leg curl combo	2	8	90

Conditioning Session: Med ball complex
1. Med ball chest pass against wall   3x5
2. Med ball side tosses against wall   3x5 each side
3. Med ball slams into floor   3x5
4. Med ball overhead toss against wall   3x5

Rest Intervals:
Workouts: 1-2: 120 sec
Workouts: 3-4: 100 sec
Workouts: 5-6: 90 sec

Tuesday

Foam and lacrosse ball rolling upper body:

1. Pec rolling 2x10 (LB)

2. Lat role (FR)

3. Lumbar – thoracic extensions 2x10

4. Lumbar – thoracic rolling 2x10

Mobility Drills:

1. Elastic band pull apart 2x10

2. Elastic band pulls behind head 2x10

3. Prone hand walks outs 2x5

Exercise	Sets	Reps	Rest
A. Log push press	5	6-8	120
B1 Football bar incline Press	4	4-6	120
B2 T-bar rows	4	5-7	120
C1 Band push-ups Feet elevated	3	8	75
C2 Suit case farmer Walk (1-arm)	3	40 yards 2-3 trips per hand	75

Wednesday

Complete recovery

Thursday

Foam rolling lower body:
1. Quadriceps
2. Hamstrings
3. TFL
4. Calfs

Mobility Drills:
1. Ankle Mobs 2x5
2. Squat to stand 2x5
3. High knee walk forward lunge 2x5
4. Kneeling rock backs 2x10

Exercise	Sets	Reps	Rest
A. Rack deadlift bar Below knee off pins	5	5-7	120
B1 Db walking lunges	4	5-7 reps per leg	100
B2 Standing leg curl	4	5-7 reps per leg	100
C1 Prowler Push **(180lb)**	3	30 yards	100
C2 Sled backwards drag **(250lb)**	3	30 yards	100

Friday

**Foam and lacrosse ball
rolling upper body:**   **Mobility Drills:**

1. Pec rolling 2x10 (LB)   1. Elastic band pull apart 2x10

2. Lat role (FR)   2. Elastic band pulls behind head 2x10

3. Lumbar – thoracic   3. Prone hand walks outs 2x5
extensions 2x10

4. Lumbar – thoracic rolling 2x10

Exercise	Sets	Reps	Rest
A. Medball explosive Chest pass against wall	5	5	5
B1. Db incline Alternating chest press	4	4-6	100
B2. Fat grip neutral grip Pull up **(weighted)**	4	4-6	100
C1. Kettlebell front Swings (2 hands)	3	6-8	75
C2. Prone 3 point row	3	6-8	75

PHASE 3: HIGH PERFORMANCE COMPLEX # 1

Days per Week: 3

Length: 6 weeks

High performance training can be a fun way to improve speed, power and strength endurance capabilities. In this phase we will begin utilizing Jonathan's new found strength by incorporating the Olympic lifts and Plyometrics that will transfer to 'on the field performance' improvement. This phase will involve training the whole body using circuits with minimal rest between exercises focusing on explosive-type movements.

Monday

Exercise	Sets	Reps	Rest
A1 Snatch Grip Deadlift	3-7	3-5	30
A2 Barbell overhead Snatch	3-7	3-5	30
A3 Broad jumps	3-7	8-10	30
A4 Barbell Jump squat @ 20% of body weight	3-7	8-10	30
A5 Sled Backwards Drag	3-7	2-3 trips @ 30 yards	90

Arm Specific Training: This would be performed after the main lifting session.

A1. Rope hammer curl 2x8-10

A2. 1-arm Barbell preacher curl 2x8-10

Rest 10 sec between exercises and 90 sec between stations

B1. Reverse cable curl 2x8-10

B2. Wide grip cable curl 2x8-10

B3. Close grip cable curl 2x8-10

Rest 10 sec between exercises and 90 sec between stations

Tuesday

Exercise	Sets	Reps	Rest
A1 Trap bar explosive Jumps	3-5	3-5	30
A2 Med ball overhead Toss **(against wall)**	3-5	3-5	30
A3 Box jumps	3-5	3-5	30
A4 Battle rope Whips	3-5	12-15	30
A5 Heavy Kettlebell Swings **(2 hands)**	3-5	12-15	90

Thursday

Exercise	Sets	Reps	Rest
A1 Power Clean	3-5	3-5	30
A2 Depth jumps For height	3-5	5	30
A3 Plyo push-ups	3-5	3-5	30
A4 Explosive Lateral Hops	3-5	8-10	30
A5 Prowler explosive Throws (in a crouch position behind the prowler, explosively push it away from you trying to create as much space as possible).	3-5	5	90

Agility Specific Training: This would be performed after the main lifting session.

1. 5-10-5 3x

2. 20 yard shuttle run 3x

FINAL TESTING RESULTS AFTER 15 WEEKS OF STRENGTH AND CONDITIONING

Day 1

1. Height: **6'4"**

2. Weight: **215lb**

3. Body Composition: **17.8%**

4. Power Clean: (1rm) **200lb**

5. Box squat (1rm) **285lb**

6. Bench Press (1rm) **225lb**

Day 2

1. Vertical Jump: **27"**

2. Med Ball Overhead Toss: **32'11"**

3. Standing Med Ball Chest Launch: **22'**

4. T-test: **8.23 sec**

5. 5-10-5: **4.6 sec**

6. 300 yard shuttle: **1:17 sec**

In conclusion, this chapter was written to give you (the coach) the best of practical experience and science. Jonathan was an average athlete who performed at a higher level his senior year because he worked harder at his physical preparation. That's what made him a better football player.

My goal in writing this chapter was to give you and your team the best training program possible – free of the fluff that does nothing but waste your time.

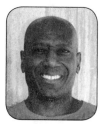

About Richard

Richard Bell, BS, CSCS, IYCA Certified High School Strength and Conditioning Coach is currently working as a High School Strength Coach in the Evergreen and Lakewood Colorado area. Richard is a highly sought after coach for athletes ages 13 and older from Junior High School to the College ranks. He also works with individuals — whether executives or stay-at-home moms — who want enhanced health and stamina, and to improve their physical appearance.

Bell's focus over the past 16 years has been to incorporate new techniques that ensure fast results, increased stamina and better performance — methods determined entirely by each athlete's personalized assessment.

Bell is a native of Boston, Massachusetts where he was a four-year starter on his high school basketball team and where he won two state championships. Rich attended the University of Maine at Farmington, where he also played Basketball and majored in Community Health Education with a concentration in Sports Conditioning. After graduating, Bell moved to the Evergreen, CO area with the vision of becoming one of the best in the strength and conditioning field.

From 2006-2009, Rich ran and operated Rich Barbell Fitness and Sports Conditioning, a performance enhancement facility located in Golden, Colorado. Rich is determined to improve the way athletes approach their strength and conditioning goals. He believes strongly in applying scientifically-proven techniques to enhance human performance on the playing field.

A large percentage of the last 10 years of Rich's life has been consumed by an overwhelming drive to better understand the true nature of improving human performance. In his early years as a Strength and Conditioning Coach, Rich worked as the Head Basketball Coach for Platte Canyon High in Bailey, Colorado. There he oversaw all his athletes' off-season weight training sessions, and this experience led him to pursue his passion for improved sports performance on a full-time basis.

Since those early days of coaching Basketball, Rich has trained over 300 athletes from various sports backgrounds and different levels.

(Rich would like to personally thank Wendy Schott of Wendy Schott Photography, for making time to work with him on his photo.)

CHAPTER 16

Metabolic Conditioning for Strength and Power

A quicker, simpler path to a better athletic fitness and performance

By Phil Hueston, NASM-PES, IYCA-YFS

In 2004, I had the opportunity to work with a young man who was a club and high school hockey player. James' hands were gifted, his skating was terrific, his ice vision was great and he possessed excellent playmaking ability.

His problem: he needed to be bigger, faster and stronger. He had less than six months to make the changes needed to get him to the next level. Less than six months…with a schedule already full of practices, tournaments and other hockey-related stuff.

"Skeptical" described his parents upon hearing from me that all we needed was 3 hours a week in the gym, and another hour a week or so outside the gym to accomplish his goals. James had been told "how to train for hockey" by several of his hockey coaches, none of whom had professional experience as youth fitness trainers. Their "prescription" included heavy bench presses, seated leg presses and miles and miles of distance running to "strengthen his legs."

I asked James a question that changed his and his parents' perspective on training, …two questions, really. I asked him if he liked his "training programs." He said "No, they take too much time. I keep skipping days and stuff." Then I asked James, "What if you did? Would you be more likely to stick to it?"

Fast forward six months: James had gained 16 pounds, improved his speed on and off skates and saw dramatic improvement in strength and power. Five months later, he was named Player of the Year by the Asbury Park Press as a *sophomore* and went on to play on the Team USA Under-17 and Under-18 teams, and was given a scholarship to play hockey at Division I Univ. of New Hampshire. In 2007, he was the 2nd overall pick in the NHL Entry Draft.

I've learned immensely from James and the thousands of other athletes like him that I've been blessed to work with over the years. Now, with over thirteen years in the Youth and Sports Fitness industry, I've noticed two key things about most "performance training programs" being offered:

1. **They take far too much time** – schedule time on a week-to-week basis, time per session and time spent in the athlete's life. Your programs need to become more than just another required block of time in the life of your youth athletes. You do this partly through quality coaching, an art form that seems absent in many Youth Fitness Pros, even some of you reading this right now.

   Most of the effectiveness of programming comes from the blending of art and science that is Metabolic Conditioning for Strength and Power.

2. **They're B-O-R-I-N-G!** Sets and reps? Learning progressions? Skill acquisition models? Training responses relative to age-related neural plasticity and peak height velocity? Really? That might be important to you and me, but the average teenager doesn't walk in to your facility thinking "How do I best maximize frontal plane knee

stabilization during the drive phase of my barbell squat? And how do I account for the variables in my neural plasticity and excitability created by the stresses of failing a test and getting dumped by my boyfriend/girlfriend?"

Many of you dream of applying high-tech training techniques to those elite athletes you see walking through your doors every day, and your facilities are just overflowing with high draft choices, Division I scholarship winners and Olympians, right?

WRONG! Reality check - the bulk of our clients are NOT these people and even if they were, all the science and high tech gadgets in the world can't replace challenging programs and plain old hard work.

Your clients are *kids first* and athletes second. These kids will do anything you ask of them as long as they see the value of it, recognize the importance of it and feel that they are enjoying the process. In other words, they'll do it ...**if it doesn't SUCK!**

All the advances in strength, speed and power training, injury prevention, nutrition and other critical areas are important. Learn, remember and be able to communicate to average people the "smart stuff" like kinetic chain alignment, neuro-muscular optimization, neural plasticity, proprioception, local and global muscular activation and skill acquisition.

But none of it means a thing if your athletes and parents look at your programs and think, "This can be done at McFitness Big Box Gym for $19.99 a month." Your programs need to be effective, unique, memorable and high energy! And it wouldn't hurt you to make them fun, too, would it? *Newsflash*- **If your clients hate working out with you, they ain't coming back!**

There are four things we must address, globally, as Youth and Sports Fitness Professionals, if we are to move our industry into a new, more positive and effective realm:

1. **The glaring need for today's athletes to be stronger, faster and *to have a significantly higher capacity for work than their predecessors*.** Additionally, they must be able to continually improve that capacity, concurrent with any improvements made in strength, power, speed, agility or other aspects of what I call "the athletic skill set."

Coaches tell us, in equal measure, of the need for players to have "quick strike" ability (power & speed) *and* to "wear down their opponents (strength & endurance)." Quick strike capability is the ability to obliterate a tree with a lightning strike. Wearing down an opponent is the process of a river grinding a canyon through the countryside. One happens instantaneously - flash of blinding, focused and all-consuming energy; the other takes place as constant, grinding force is applied to erode away the ability to resist that force. Giving both capabilities to athletes requires a unique programming style.

2. **A decreased time availability and competition for attention.** Today's athletes, particularly student-athletes, have more time demands and distractions than any generation before them. Sure, some of these are "voluntary" in nature but we must recognize this fact nonetheless. In order to serve our "tribe," the student-athletes, we must become more effective shamans as it relates to the "magic" of our sports fitness and performance programs.

Realities of time stress for kids, especially athletes, include their scholastic sports, homework, club/rec sports, jobs, requirements at home (babysitting, chores, etc.), dating and social events, and "tech time." *Tech time* is the phrase I use to refer to time spent texting one another, time spent on social media or surfing the internet and time spent playing video games.

These voluntary time "wasters" are simply a part of life to the average student-athlete. Put aside your opinion about them and get down to the business of helping student-athletes manage time through the improvement of our programming relative to their time demands.

3. **The struggle between "more is better" or "cooler/higher tech is better" and the truth of "Better Is Better."** Long, grueling workouts used to be the hallmark of "great" and "tough" sports fitness trainers. Vomiting was part of the normal course of a "great session." Not being able to walk/comb your hair/shampoo your head was a sign that you had "trashed" whatever body part you victimized the previous day.

There was virtually no thought about improvements to speed and agility, mobility, flexibility, stability and injury prevention or whether the athlete developed or reinforced any critical movement skills. Why? Because the trainers involved didn't know better. The ones who still train that way are Neanderthals and should be drummed out of the industry. The same goes for the "high-speed" or "over-speed" treadmill crowd. Seriously...high-speed treadmills? Idiotic!

Let me be clear: athletes run on the ground and push off of (mostly) non-moving surfaces. They push and pull against other athletes and against objects and implements, many of which are unstable and require control. All of this takes place in a chaotic, multi-directional, multi-dimensional, multi-speed environment under intense time and performance pressure. They require levels of dynamic strength and power, kinesthetic differentiation, spatial awareness and multi-directional movement capabilities that cannot be acquired while sitting or lying down on a bench or "spinning their wheels" on an over-speed treadmill.

So do you really think lying on a bench, pushing dead weight off your chest will improve performance under those conditions? How about pushing too much weight, usually with abysmal form, up and down several hundred times in the exact same (insufficient) range of motion and movement pattern until you "trash" the muscles involved? How about "running" on a treadmill while your idiot trainer talks to you about "ramping it up?" Let me help you with that: NO! Because NONE of them look anything like sports!

4. **"Want to" or "get to" vs. "have to." Or, the fun factor!** Athletes, and ESPECIALLY if you want to work with "non" athletes or casual youth athletes, will never respond to you and your programming until you change their perspective from one of "I **HAVE** to go to training" to one of "Awesome! I'm going to see Coach _____!!" Create a training environment that emphasizes the reasons they like to play sports in the first place: 1). They're FUN, and 2). Athletes (and all kids, to some degree) are competitive by nature. Even those kids who "don't like organized sports" will be willing to work on a team during a training session if you program in some fun!

So, then, how do we create this multi-disciplinary, multi-modality revolution in training systems in order to address the needs of our youth athletes?

Within each session and cycle of programming, we must address flexibility, mobility, joint stabilization, local and global muscle activation, core stability, core strength and core power, systemic strength, movement skill acquisition and improvement, cardio-respiratory capacity improvement, local system strength improvement and integration of local muscle systems into a unified force production/reduction system.

It's also important to provide regressions and progressions for each exercise we choose in order to ensure that our athletes develop and progress, regardless of their current or starting developmental level.

Session structure can vary based on any number of variables, the simplest being a desire to create variety over a given period in order to keep the athletes motivated and interested. I'll offer two model sessions here, one integrated sports fitness session, including a MetCon Challenge, and one Athletic Circuit Training session.

For more information about Metabolic Conditioning for Strength and Power and more sample workouts, go to my website www.allstarsportsacademynj.com/metconsp

SESSION 1

Warm-up (All X 2):

Carioca	20 yards each direction
Overhead Lunge/jog	20 yards
Skip with big arm circles	2 x 20 yards
Iron Cross	6/leg
Scorpion	6/leg
Kneeling Hip Flexor stretch	20 sec hold, 2/leg

Phase 1 (3 rounds, 30 sec/30 sec work/rest ratio):

Barbell or Dumbbell Romanian Dead Lift

Med Ball high arc 1/2 sit-up rotations

TRX Pike

Kettlebell alternating crunch press (floor-based rolling "crunch" movement w/KB push towards ceiling)

Phase 2 (the Challenge):

MetCon Challenge - finish all the listed work in 15 minutes or less. Complete the work using any order/breakdown you choose:

20 yard sprint (2) to Kettlebell swings (10)   6 rounds total

SAQ Ladder shuffle (in-in-out) to reverse shuffle (1 each way) 6 rounds total

Slide "Hand Runners"   60 total reps
(We use ValSlides. One on each hand in push-up position. Slide both at once in opposite directions in the sagittal plane. Each double hand movement is one rep.)

Hurdle 2-4   8 total in each direction (16)

Rope slams (2 arm, any style)   80 total reps

Prowler Push (power sled) 100 lbs total load, 20 yards
10 total passes

TRX Mountain Climber   80 total reps

SESSION 2 – ATHLETIC CIRCUIT TRAINING

12 stations, work-to-rest ratios can vary from 1:1 to 3:1, depending on athlete conditioning levels and types of exercises employed. I recommend longer rest periods if Olympic lifts or variants are being used, to allow for proper set-up and prep for each athlete.

Suggestions for accommodating varying strength levels with barbell exercises, TRX training and bodyweight exercises:

1. Set up several barbells with different weights and/or at different rack heights to allow different athletes to quickly access age- or level-appropriate weights.

2. Where possible, have bands or chains available for stronger athletes to increase weight or load quickly without a long breakdown time between stations. Anchor bands to heavy dumbbells, squat racks or kettlebells.

3. Keep a light weighted vest (10 – 20 lbs) near your TRX units so stronger athletes can easily increase the load for pull-ups/rows, push-ups and other TRX exercises.

4. For push-ups, overhead presses, battle ropes and kettlebell swings, use "players choice," thereby allowing athletes to progress to higher difficulty or skill level variations of

commonly used exercises. Coach wisely to prevent over-reaching!

Warm-up: Use a movement-based warm up similar to that of Session 1....(5 – 7 minutes)

Sample Session; 3 rounds – 1st round - 40 seconds of work, 20 seconds of rest; rounds 2 & 3 – 30:30

1. Plank Up – move from stable plank position to push up position and back with minimal hip rotation
2. Jump Rope (players choice)
3. TRX squat to row (SL leg rounds 1(rt.) & 2 (left), 2 leg round 3)
4. Band-resisted forward/backward Bear Crawl – anchor bands firmly
5. Barbell Squat – offer dumbbell squat for those new to squatting or to your program
6. Speed Ladder shuffle or crossover shuffle – offer reverse movement as an option
7. Standing barbell/dumbbell Overhead Press
8. Stability ball bridge with medicine ball overhead extension – scapula stable, arms moving overhead with med ball
9. Lateral hurdles – use 4-6 hurdles
10. Push up – players choice
11. Battle rope slams – players choice
12. Prowler or power sled push – Have 10 – 20 lb dumbbells available to quickly add load if needed

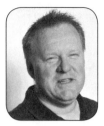

About Phil

Phil Hueston is the co-owner of All-Star Sports Academy and Co-Head Coach at Athletic Revolution – Toms River, NJ. He has been, and continues to be, a sought after Sports Performance Trainer and Consultant to teams and athletes at the Youth Sports, high school, collegiate and professional levels.

Since his entrance into the fitness industry in 1998, he has questioned the *status quo*, challenged the conventional wisdom of the fitness industry and used the answers to make his clients better, bigger, faster and stronger.

Not just another pretty trainer, Phil has been called a "master motivator and trainer of high school athletes" and a "key player in the Youth Fitness industry." He works with athletes, "mathletes" and "non-letes" from 6 to 18, helping them all reach their performance potential and maximize their "fun quotient."

Phil recognized early on that the ONLY task of Sports Fitness Professionals is *the improvement of their clients' sports performance and their enjoyment of the process!* He has worked with 1000's of athletes; he's assisted them on their journeys to collegiate sports, Division 1 scholarships, pro and semi-pro sports careers and even the first round of the NHL Draft.

To learn more about Phil Hueston and his groundbreaking training system *"Metabolic Conditioning for Strength and Power,"* visit: www.allstarsport-sacademynj.com/metconsp and don't forget to request your free report *"21 MetCon Workouts for Strength & Power."*

CHAPTER 17

From Homemade to Hoboken Bootcamp

By David Cabral

What does a kid growing up in Brooklyn do if he wants to work out and can't afford to join a gym? If that kid is David Cabral, he not only builds his own gym but, in the process, creates an entirely new approach to exercise which, years later, will change the way the country looks at getting and staying physically fit.

David Cabral has mastered turning obstacles into opportunities. He discovered his passion for exercise during that Brooklyn childhood. When he realized that there would be no gym membership and no trainer, he turned his mother's garage into his personal work out studio.

"I had to be creative. I had to invent my own equipment and my own exercise routine," David recalls.

And invent he did. Everyday household items became his exercise equipment. One gallon, plastic milk containers filled with sand became dumb bells. Tossing stones back and forth in the yard and carrying heavy bags of laundry became part of his daily exercise routine. He jogged to city parks where he used benches and jungle gyms as part of his ever-expanding workout world. He did push ups wherever he found the space.

Before long, David stopped wishing for a gym membership, because he had discovered the challenge and the joy of creating his own workout routine with his self- designed equipment. He also soon started noticing the results of his daily workouts.

"I'm a big guy and lifting weights seemed like something I was always supposed to do," David remarks – when telling of those early workouts in his mother's garage in New Jersey, and in that storage unit he rented to use as his own underground workout studio.

When asked how he knew that he was 'supposed to be lifting weights and working out' and how, ultimately, he also knew that he was supposed to help others learn methods of increasing their personal fitness, David is not able to put that awareness into words.

"It's just something I felt. Something I knew. Some sort of inner drive leading me to what I consider my destiny."

Coming from someone else, that statement might sound like someone too full of self-importance to formulate a reasonable response to a reasonable question. However, David Cabral is far from being full of himself or from feeling full of his own self-importance. He is a humble man who accepts a life task he did not seek.

"I didn't go looking for this. It just sort of found me."

As David pursued his own exercise goals he began to also consider how he might help others become more physically fit without having to join expensive gyms. He toyed with various ideas until his son was born.

"Then I knew I had to get serious. I had to stop toying with ideas and make something happen. Having a son to raise and support changed my focus." David merged his love of exercise, his desire to help others achieve higher levels of physical fitness, and his need to financially support his son into the creation of Hoboken's 35-Minute Boot camps and his 35-Minute Workout.

The Bootcamps' studio in Hoboken has all of the ambience of a Brooklyn garage. It is filled with equipment – some purchased and much created – and also filled with energy and laughter. Workouts aren't confined to the inside of the studio. Much like he used the streets and parks of his childhood Brooklyn for his gym, David and his coaches use loading ramps and steps and ladders inside and outside to provide opportunities for participants to learn and practice daily fitness. One participant remembers a particular exercise session, during which David led the group in moving boxes of newly delivered Kettlebells from one side of the studio to the other. Another participant tells of a session spent running up and down flights of stairs. Yet another participant laughs about the session in which she ran while lifting a tire up over her head and then lowering it to hold it around her waist. "I kept telling myself that it was only for thirty-five minutes – that it couldn't possibly last forever."

When asked about these unusual workout sessions, David replies, "I wanted them to realize that good workouts can happen anyplace using whatever we have. The boxes of Kettlebells had just been delivered and they needed to be moved around – probably not as much as they got moved but no one complained. And the tires? Well, you gotta do something with old tires. Why not turn them into exercise equipment? And stairs are just begging to become part of a workout routine."

Clearly for David Cabral, that Brooklyn and New Jersey workout style remains an important part of his life. Not only does he not want to forget it, he wants his participants to also think of that playground, garage, and storage unit.

"That garage training was the best thing for me. I learned to be creative. No, I had to be creative if I wanted to lift weights and move forward. Now I want to help others feel that creativity. And I want the children who attend classes at the studio to develop a sense of appreciation for the simple, everyday things in their lives. That's what I want for my son, so why wouldn't I want it for all the kids in my life. This type of training and thinking helps us build toughness – both physical and mental. We need that to help us live. Isn't that why we exercise to begin with?"

Even though he continues to use some home-made equipment and even though his approach to exercise is his own, David became a certified personal trainer because he knew certification would add validity to his creative approaches. He has been certified for more than six years.

His first certification is as a National Academy of Sports Medicine Trainer. Since 1987, the National Academy of Sports Medicine (NASM) has provided evidence-based certifications. The mission of that organization is to provide health and fitness professionals with a variety of evidence-based systems for exercises and workouts. David didn't need that type of certification to provide evidence that his approach to working out is effective. All he had to do was ask the people who attend his 35 Minute Boot camp studio. Nevertheless, at the time certification was important to David.

David then became an Underground Strength Coach by Zach Even-Esh. This was where David learned how to put all his passion for fitness and untraditional training all together. He learned that it takes action, heart, and hard work to be the best. After this certification, David's mission was clear. He knew that he wanted to make an impact on every child and adult looking to live a fit lifestyle. He wants to help his members reach their maximum potential both physically and mentally.

He also holds several certifications for Kettlebell workouts. He is certified by the International Kettlebell and Fitness Federation. A Kettlebell is a cast-iron weight looking a lot like a cannonball with a handle attached. Using a Kettlebell in a workout routine combines cardiovascular, strength training and flexibility training. Unlike traditional dumbbells, a Kettlebell's center goes beyond the hand holding it. Its shape encourages swinging movements.

"Kettlebells are great for building strength and endurance especially in the lower back and shoulders. Their use mimics real world activities such as shoveling snow," David explains. He goes on to say the one of the reasons he chooses Kettlebells is because of their similarity in movement and workout to ordinary activities. David became certified in their use to, once again, formalize and validate his unique approach to work out. Part of that unique approach is David's belief that getting into shape can be compared to a child learning to walk. The baby crawls before getting up and running. "People beginning to exercise need to start with the basics."

David is committed to helping people begin with simple and effective routines. He talks to his Bootcamp participants in plain language and assures them that they can meet their goals. Because of his approach, the Bootcamp participants not only meet their goals, but also set new goals and achieve them. David reminds participants that, "I am 100% committed to your health. Give me 35 minutes and I'll give you real results."

Cabral easily shares his approach to fitness by encouraging participants to use their own garage-made exercise equipment — broom sticks, soccer balls, tennis balls, sand bags, jump ropes. He encourages participants to play 'no equipment needed' games such as tug of war with jump ropes. He loves browsing in hardware stores to find more tools he can turn into exercise equipment. Anything can be a workout, you just have to know how to use it and stay safe. A common piece of Home Depot workout equipment is heavy chains. Standing with a tow chain at your feet and lifting it overhead for a few reps really works your arms and core. And fifteen feet of Grade A alloy chain is cheaper than a few dumb bells any day. Sand bags are also a favorite of his. Throw a forty-five pound bag of sand over your shoulders and start doing squats and lunges and you have yourself a full body workout.

"We should all be able to work out without breaking the bank," Cabral says. One would understandably wonder how long a workout studio, which encourages its participants to make their own equipment or use whatever they find around the house to create their own exercises, can stay in business.

"Our Bootcamp studio," Cabral explains, " is nothing fancy. We don't have showers and we don't have lockers. Here's what we are. We're a place for people to come and spend a little over half-an-hour learning their own potentials. They get a lot of exercise in a nothing fancy studio with other people and come only because they want to achieve their highest physical potential. And then they leave for work or home or grocery shopping or child care. They leave sweaty and smiling."

David doesn't worry about his clients realizing they no longer need 35 Minute Bootcamps. "If they don't need us because they've figured out how to do it on their own, that's great. But even if they do figure that out, doing this type of stuff on your own isn't nearly as much fun as doing it with other people trying as hard as you are, and staff coaching and encouraging and praising. And don't forget. We're all about fun."

While he started out on his own, these days David doesn't do any of this by himself. He has assembled a team of teachers, coaches and manager who work with him, keep him focused, nag him, and remind him of his original vision. The studio is now more than a place to workout. Participants can study yoga and talk about healthy eating choices. The studio is available for events such as parties and presentations. And, of course, David and his staff offer something for all ages – even, or especially, for children.

Clearly David Cabral is passionate about his own exercises, about helping others with their exercises and about modeling healthy living for his son – who is now old enough to frequently visit the Boot Camp studio. "My son sees me constantly working out. I am setting an example for him. He started trying to flip small tires and lift heavy rocks – heavy for him, that is. Pretty soon he was doing push ups with me. He wanted to do everything I was doing. I made him some sand bags to lift. Now he's five years old and he spends a lot of time at the studio. It's like a little playground for him. He does push ups and climbs walls and just has fun."

Indeed, the experience of David's son seems very similar to the experiences of those who attend the studio workshops. They climb walls and move equipment and jump through tires and lunge across the parking lot and laugh and have fun. And that's pretty much what David Cabral envisioned when he opened his Bootcamp studio.

Recognizing that time and money are precious, he asks people to spend little of either on their workouts. Thirty-five minutes, in fact, is all the time he asks because just about anyone can spare that much time. "With that amount of time," he proposes, "a person can sculpt muscles, improve strength and gain more energy than ever imagined." He also promises that – with creativity developed in Brooklyn – no two classes will ever be alike.

"With a little creativity, all things are possible. Athletic training does not have to come from a high-end facility. It comes from the will and the drive to be better than the rest. All I have to do is give people the tools and teach them how to perform."

With a little creativity all things are possible and just because you don't have, doesn't mean you can't. That statement sums up the approach to life David brings from Brooklyn to Hoboken, and on to wherever his vision leads him. Indeed, with creativity born in Brooklyn in his mother's garage and that small storage unit in NJ, David Cabral is changing the way people go about the business of becoming more physically fit.

To find out more please visit: www.35minutebootcamps.com

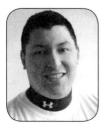

About David

David C. Cabral has been a certified personal trainer for more than six years. He is also a Kettlebell Certified Coach and an Underground Strength Coach. David has been running boot camps in New Jersey and New York City for nearly three.

Cabral's personal belief is that getting into shape is like a child learning to walk; a baby needs to crawl before he gets up and runs! He is deeply committed to teaching and guiding exercisers through his simple, effective routines.

His expertise is in mastering new workout techniques and teaching those techniques to his 'bootcampers' in plain language, guaranteeing that every fitness level will be served, from the "work-out queen" to the "couch potato."

Cabral uses a combination of body weight exercises, kettlebells, sandbags, medicine balls, stretch bands and calisthenics in short circuits for time, reps and rounds. He keeps your muscles guessing (and strengthening) by "mixing it up"!

"I am 100% committed to your health. Give me 35 minutes and I'll give you real results."

David Cabral - Owner/ Founder
www.35minutebootcamps.com

CHAPTER 18

DIAMOND IN THE ROUGH

By Cory Skillin

I want you to reflect for a moment: think of all the coaches you've had throughout your life. Start with pee wee sports and work your way up to the present. How many names do you remember? How many of those special people had a positive impact not only on your life as an athlete but also on the person you've become?

For me, I can say I've learned something important from every coach I've ever had. Some were capital motivators who helped forge my character by teaching me commitment and dedication through hard work and perseverance. Some were masters of technique; whether it involved weight training, a cover-two defense, or conditioning, these people taught me the intricacies of athletic processes and how mastering these things translated into being a successful athlete. Others got the best out of me by providing positive feedback; they had a knack for knowing when I needed an encouraging word rather than a 'kick in the ass.' But the best coaches I studied under utilized all of these approaches when plying their craft. This isn't easy. But that's the ideal I strive for when I coach: a synthesis of all of the best attributes possessed by the coaches that taught me over the years.

I believe coaches need this multi-faceted approach, because we encounter so many different temperaments and personalities. We can't employ a one-size-fits-all model, because our effectiveness is often dependent upon our ability to recognize the best way to motivate and instruct a given athlete, and all athletes are not the same.

I've been a competitor since I was a kid. I was a little brother! So not a day went by without some type of contest. I'd play all kinds of games and sports with him and his friends. Didn't matter what we were doing—soccer, football, baseball, capture the flag, twenty-one, whatever—it was a fierce competition. Being the smallest and youngest, I learned I had to work twice as hard as everyone else just to survive. But, in the long run, going up against bigger, faster kids made me a better athlete.

When I got into high school, I started weight training with my football team. The program our team followed was a cookie cutter, one-size-fits-all method for high school athletes. This program had a national ranking system for athletes that could move a certain amount of weight for selected exercises. The emphasis to get more players on the record board resulted in poor training technique.

Going into my last year of high school football, I had 'trained my ass off.' Completed each and every workout given. I felt like I was in great shape, but a few weeks into the season I started experiencing severe back pain. As the season went on, the pain got worse, to the point where I was forced to skip drills and eventually sat out some practices—not a situation you want to be in when you are a team captain in your senior year. I was unable to play in some of my final high school games. When I look back on it, I believe the injuries I sustained can be traced to poor weight training technique.

I was not offered a scholarship or recruited to play college football. But I was encouraged by a close friend to try out for our college team. So I walked on the team during the offseason. This gave me a great opportunity to get to know my teammates and try to make an impression on my coaches.

The strength and conditioning program we used was an exact duplicate of a popular one used by a large university at the time. Since we didn't have an actual strength and conditioning coach, there wasn't any real technical instruction. I learned how to lift from my teammates. This program was much better than the one I'd followed in high school but still far from perfect. Like the high school program, the emphasis was on how much weight you could move. There weren't any coaches to correct you if you did something wrong. The only supervision involved checking us in, making sure we completed our workout, and recording our numbers for the day.

I worked hard and performed well enough to get invited to pre-season camp. When I got there, I was unceremoniously placed on the look team right smack at the bottom of the depth chart! This was humbling, but it turned out to be a blessing. My role was to prepare the first-string offense for upcoming opponents. I had to cover two all-American wide receivers everyday. This allowed me to hone my skills and develop my own style of playing defensive back. I was able to try different techniques and see what worked best in different situations. My game progressed more during this time than ever before—trial by error! It ultimately earned me a spot in the starting lineup.

I played four years of college football and was lucky enough to escape without any major surgeries. Other than a broken wrist and a couple of sprained ankles, I was injury free. Even so, the few injuries I sustained required quite a bit of rehab, and I learned a lot through the process that has helped me in my career as a coach.

My senior year, our school hired a new Head Athletic Trainer. She came from a big Division I University in the Midwest. She was a force: energetic, hands on, with an incredible amount of athletic knowledge. Right away, she helped me with the nagging back injury that had bothered me since high school. After a few tests, she surmised that my trouble derived from a weak trunk. I had not been exposed to any core training up to that point—it simply hadn't been part of any of the programs I'd followed. But after I incorporated a core strength component into my workouts, my back trouble ceased.

Working with athletes while interning with this woman during the offseason is what inspired me to become a strength and conditioning coach. I was fascinated by all of the things she taught me. My own body had started to feel a lot better after implementing some simple exercises she suggested. It was a revealing experience for me. I was blown away by how much a person could positively impact another's health and athletic potential with good information and training methods. I thought it was the coolest stuff in the world, and it made me wonder how good my team could have been if we'd trained under her watch for four years.

Before any athlete tested for certain lifts, she made them perform the movements with little or no load. This seemed silly to many of the athletes—find someone on a football team who wants to be seen performing a lift with no weight on the bar or, God forbid, a wooden dowel in place of a bar! I witnessed many studs eating huge pieces of humble pie as they attempted to perform Olympic lifts with broom sticks. It was fascinating to watch a guy who could squat a house lack the mobility and core strength to perform an unloaded overhead squat or hold a basic plank.

This taught me that when you coach someone for the first time, no matter how big or strong they seem, you have to start them with the basics. You have to see your athletes move with your own eyes—you can't take their word for it! More isn't always better: sometimes it's necessary to back off and regress a movement. This can be a hard thing to convince athletes to do. Watching this lady demonstrate how to properly execute each and every exercise or agility drill she required was something I really admired. She wasn't operating in a vacuum or ordering people to do some esoteric thing while she sat and watched. She was involved and could do everything she asked of her athletes. I was extremely impressed by how easy she made things look.

Looking back on my athletic career I can't help but remember all of the teammates I had who either quit playing for various reasons or were forced to stop because of injuries. It makes me think that with the proper attention, many of these situations could have been prevented.

But it's not just injuries that can force someone out of athletics. I made the decision to play football in high school when I no longer enjoyed playing soccer. I loved soccer, but I had a coach who just took the fun out of it. Have you ever had a coach who caused you to have a negative experience with a sport you once loved? Or have you sustained injuries caused by improper training you learned at a young age? Or maybe you had a coach overlook you because you weren't the fastest or strongest kid on your team? Do you feel like you missed your opportunity to be one of the next great phenoms because you weren't exposed to the proper training? Sadly, there are situations like these happening everyday all over the world.

Quitting athletics, for me, would have been something that haunted me for the rest of my life. That's the major reason I chose to try to walk on and play college football. Despite what my high school coach thought, I felt like I could compete at a college level and contribute to a team. If I'd followed my high school coach's advice, I would have missed out on four of the most rewarding years of my life. I try to remember all of these things when I coach today—I don't want to be the reason someone never realized a dream.

HERE ARE MY TOP FIVE TIPS TO BEING A GREAT YOUTH CONDITIONING COACH

(1) Never stop educating yourself. You owe it to your youth athletes to provide them with the very best information and methods available. If you aren't keeping up, you're falling behind. The International Youth Conditioning Association (www.IYCA.org) is the gold standard for youth athletic development and fitness, and

I suggest you start there: attend a seminar or watch a training DVD. But that's just the tip of a huge iceberg: there are endless sources of information that can make you a better youth conditioning coach.

(2) Lead by example. How can you expect your athletes to buy into what you're trying to teach them if you don't follow your own rules and suggestions? What you do impacts kids more than what you say: you can't tell them one thing and do the opposite. Your athletes will look to you for guidance if you do what you say. They will respect you for it.

(3) Evaluate your athletes' movement. If you evaluate basic movements, you can determine where to start with your program design for a given athlete. Assuming things rarely works out. By performing basic screens, you can ascertain where you need to start someone's journey of developing into a great athlete.

(4) Keep an empathetic attitude. Remember what it's like to be a kid. Regardless of what age group you're working with, try to look at things from their point of view. Remember all of the outside stress you experienced growing up—it isn't always the easiest time in someone's life: peer pressure, family issues, tests at school, boyfriends, girlfriends, not to mention the emotional and hormonal changes your body undergoes, all of these things can impact a kid's athletic acumen. You are there to lift up your athletes, not beat them down.

(5) Be inspirational. Strive to make each kid that comes through your door a better person. Know that because you've coached a kid, he or she will have skills to help them on and off the field for the rest of their lives. Something as simple as a pat on the head, a high five, or a few words of encouragement can be life changing. You may be the only person in their young life that gives them positive feedback. Be in the youth conditioning business not only to make kids better athletes but to make them better people. You want to be the coach they look back on one day and say, "That person changed my life!"

Cory Skillin
Denver, CO
303 330 3868

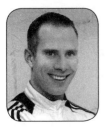

About Cory

Cory Skillin holds a Bachelor of Science degree in Physical Education, Health and Fitness from Plymouth State University where he played four years of football. Cory is also a Certified Strength and Conditioning Specialist with the National Strength and Conditioning Association, a Level 2 Junior Coach with Titleist Performance Institute, a Youth Conditioning Specialist with the International Youth Conditioning Association, and also a Certified Personal Trainer with the American Council on Exercise. Cory is changing lives each and every day in Denver, Colorado.

He can be reached at: coryskillin@yahoo.com.

CHAPTER 19

Six Strategies For Preventing ACL Injuries Among High School Female Athletes

By Timothy M. Rudd

Anterior Cruciate Ligament (ACL) injuries have become common place in young athletes participating in jumping and cutting sports, especially among high school female athletes. Females are eight more times likely to have an ACL injury compared to their male counterparts. There are 100,000 ACL injuries per year in which 30,000 are high school-aged female athletes. ACL Injuries are on the rise, nearing epidemic proportions.

There is plenty of research that suggests several reasons for the higher incidence of these injuries among the female athletes. Some cite the anatomical differences such as a wider hip angle, narrower femoral notch, strength imbalances, altered muscle recruitment patterns, faulty running patterns and jumping techniques, and even menstrual status. Now of course, not much can be done about the hormonal differences, but when we look at the other factors, we begin to understand how vital a good training program that addresses these issues is in reducing this high incidence of ACL injuries among female athletes.

The majority of ACL injuries are non-contact injuries. They typically involve a position of slight knee flexion (less than 30 degrees) coupled with *valgus* loading of the knee (caving inward), and external rotation of the foot relative to the *tibia* (foot turned out). They almost always occur on one foot in a diagonal pattern. This is important to understand when developing an effective ACL injury prevention/reduction program.

The sad fact is that many young athletes are exposed to bad training programs, in which coaches or trainers lack the knowledge or expertise to implement an effective training program that could have avoided many of the injuries cited above.

Basically, ACL prevention is just a good solid training program. This training program must include the following six strategies when designing and implementing an ACL injury-prevention program:

1. Active Warm-up

2. Power and Stability (Eccentric Strength)

3. Strength development on one leg

4. Change of direction concepts

5. Change of direction conditioning

6. Nutrition

Each of these strategies must be included when designing and implementing an ACL reduction program. If you just pick one or eliminate just one, you reduce the effectiveness of the program.

But before I get into the nuts and bolts of each strategy, we first must understand a misunderstood concept in our industry over the last century, and that is, Functional Training. This will be an important concept in the application of a good ACL prevention program.

When people hear the term *functional training*, most will picture people standing on Bosu balls, stability balls etc… performing circus-like exercises requiring extreme balance and stability. These exercises never will be applicable to any sport that I know of. So what is Functional Training? Well, it's the application of functional anatomy to training – which means understanding how the body works and applying these concepts to a training program.

Functional Training becomes vital to an effective ACL injury-reduction program. As I mentioned earlier, ACL injuries typically occur on one leg, so it's important to understand that everything functionally changes when we stand on one leg.

First, we have the Lateral Sub-System. The function of this system on one foot is Frontal Plane Stabilization (Lateral). The muscles included in this system are the *Glute Medius*, *Adductor Complex*, and *Quadratus Lumborum*. When an athlete stands on one foot all these muscles have to do a lot more work compared to if they were standing on two feet. The Adductor becomes a stabilizer of the Pelvis on one leg, and on the opposite, the *Quadratus Lumborum* also becomes a stabilizer of the Pelvis. So the ability of the young athlete to stabilize the Pelvis completely changes on foot. Now, this is vital when considering that the Pelvis helps to stabilize the Femur, which will help to remedy the valgus knees in weak female athletes.

Next we have the Deep Longitudinal Sub-System. The function of this system is force transmission and force production, which plays a big role in acceleration and deceleration in sport. The muscles included in this system are *Peroneals*, *Biceps Femoris*, *Sacrotuberous Ligament* and *Erect Spinae*. Basically this system comes from the ground up through the *Peroneals*, *Biceps Femoris*, *Sacrotuberous Ligament* and *Erect Spinae* up and through to the next system, *posterior*, through the core.

Finally, the *Posterior Oblique* Sub-System whose function is transverse plane (Rotational) stabilization in the Lumbar Pelvic Hip Complex (LPHC). The muscles in this system include the *Gluteus Maximus*, *Latissimus Dorsi*, and *Thoracolumbar Fascia*. Once the forces come up from the Deep Longitudinal Sub-System they transfer through the *Gluteus Maximus* then through the *Thoraco-lumbar Fascia* into the opposite side *Latissimus Dorsi.*

When athletes are on one leg, you can see that functionally there is a diagonal link posterior from the Deep Longitudinal Sub-System up to the *Posterior Oblique* Sub-system. It's important to understand these systems and their function in a single leg stance with concern to an ACL injury-reduction program.

So now that we have a better understanding of how athletes are at risk for ACL injuries, how they occur and how they function on one leg, we can then start introducing each ACL Reduction Strategy and its role in reducing the female high school athlete's chance of ACL injury.

ACL Reduction Strategy #1
GOOD ACTIVE WARM-UP

A good <u>active</u> warm-up should develop single leg strength, dynamic flexibility and proprioceptive input, all while:

1. Raising core temperature

2. Elongating muscles actively

3. Activation of proprioceptors, stabilizers and central nervous system

4. Ingrain proper motor (movement) patterns

The key to an effective warm-up is that it activates one muscle while elongating another. The warm-up should be done with a purpose and target muscles to activate, along with a target muscle to elongate.

For example in Frontal Plane (Lateral) Hip Mobility the young athlete would perform a lateral squat or lunge elongating the adductors, while activating the quads. In Saggital (Forward) Plane Hip Mobility a young athlete would perform a Split Squat or Forward Lunge activating the Quads while elongating the Hip

Flexors. Finally, in Transverse (Rotational) Hip Mobility, the athlete would perform a Hip Hinge Single Leg Dead Lift activating the Hamstring and Glute and well as elongating the Hamstrings and Glutes.

These are just some examples of exercises that should be included in a warm-up. Also, with concern to ACL injury-prevention, making sure to target muscles in all three planes of motion, which, as discussed, are vital in the stabilization of the Pelvis, and force transmission and production when on a single leg. So in short, a good warm-up is injury-prevention, which turns muscles on as well as strengthens them.

ACL Reduction Strategy #2
<u>DEVELOP STABILITY</u>

First increase eccentric strength, then eventually increase power. This would consist of a progressive plyometric program that first develops eccentric strength, then eventually progresses to power development – linearly, laterally and medially.

Phase 1: Jump or hop onto a box

1. Develop eccentric strength (stability)...

2. By developing the ability to Jump, Hop and Land

3. By minimizing gravity to improve eccentric strength

Jumping up without coming down reduces stress by reducing acceleration on the way down (produces force and reduces force).

You must hop medially and laterally. Hopping medially stresses the hip stabilizers to a greater degree than lateral hops. *Example: hopping from right leg to right leg toward midline of body is a single leg medial hop.*

Phase 2: Introduce the gravity component by jumping or hopping over a hurdle. Still focus on sticking the landing but now with a higher eccentric force. We continue to develop the young athletes eccentric strength ability.

Phase 3: Introduce the elastic component by adding a bounce in-between the hurdles. Most young athletes aren't ready at this phase to switch to a complete eccentric – to concentric loading (true Plyometrics). So we first add a bounce in this phase to introduce this component, without overloading the system. We are more concerned about rhythm of the bounce than the speed at which the athlete jumps or hops over the hurdles.

Phase 4: Now we introduce pure eccentric to concentric loading. This is now when the athlete is ready to express the stretch shortening cycle of the transition of landing to immediately jumping or hopping back up with as little foot contact time as possible. This, in its true sense, is the development of power.

So it's important to remember during these progressions that the focus is on Quality <u>over</u> Quantity. If the quality decreases with the addition of gravity, then eccentric strength is an issue. The athlete should not proceed to the next phase; in fact they should regress back to the previous phase until adequate eccentric strength is developed. In making sure that quality is never compromised, it's best to keep the volume around 25 foot contacts a day, or 100 foot contacts a week. It's best to increase intensity throughout the phases rather than volume. I should also note that in good plyometric programs, the athletes must be able to jump and land from the same position.

Following this progressive approach to power development is vital in reducing ACL injuries in young female athletes, far too often they lack the eccentric strength required for efficient cutting and landings. Most ACL injuries happen on a single leg in a diagonal pattern. So in order to reduce injuries, we need to implement training strategies that are going to mimic the mechanism of injury.

ACL Reduction Strategy #3
STRENGTH DEVELOPMENT

Young athletes must have a motor in which to produce and reduce force. Getting high school female athletes stronger is the number one line of defense in reducing the chance of an ACL injury.

If a female athlete lacks strength, especially on a single leg, then they are at high risk of injuring their ACL. Below are the progressions of an ACL injury-reduction strength program:

1. Handle bodyweight first and single leg progressions appropriately.

2. Develop functional strength. No Machines!

3. Develop single leg strength. Remember the difference in hip mechanics when athletes are on one foot.

4. Perform both knee dominant, hip dominant and hybrid single-leg exercises.

Exercise progressions will depend on each individual athlete, as every athlete should be taken through some type of screening to assess imbalances in context of stability and mobility of functional movement patterns, throughout each joint of the body. It's also important to note the athlete's chronological age as well as training age, when developing a progressive ACL reduction strength program, should also be taken into account when discussing volume and intensity.

ACL Reduction Strategy #4
CHANGE OF DIRECTION CONCEPTS

1. Teach change of direction skills.

2. Teach stable landing concepts. This is the key to injury prevention.

3. Change of direction progression:

- Stability
- Ground reaction
- Assisted-Resisted
- Transition from linear to lateral change of direction.
  Example: crossover step to linear acceleration

It is important to teach young athletes how to move better and more efficiently. Acceleration and deceleration are skills that are an integral part of most sports, and almost always occur in all three planes of motion. As I mentioned at the beginning of this article, faulty running patterns and jumping techniques were cited as major factors in ACL injuries among athletes. Far too often athletes are just mindlessly taken through drills without any teaching or skill development. So being able to break down a movement skill into parts, and explaining the how and the why of each skill and how it relates to improving on field or court performance, will go a long way in reducing ACL injuries among high school female athletes.

ACL Reduction Strategy #5
<u>CHANGE OF DIRECTION CONDITIONING</u>

Most of the time athletes will get injured when fatigued, so it's important that we teach young athletes to perform change of direction movements while under fatigue. This of course can only happen after athletes have mastered and have shown proficiency in change of direction concepts. This is another problem that happens far too often. Trainers and coaches will put young athletes through change of direction conditioning skills that were never taught. What you end up with is athletes performing change of direction skills with bad technique, which will ingrain bad movement patterns, further increasing the athlete's chance of injury.

So it's important once the athlete has been taught effectively how to change direction, that we incorporate starting and stopping into their conditioning program. This is important in minimizing injuries, and teaches them how to accelerate and decelerate under fatigue.

ACL Reduction Strategy #6
NUTRITION

This usually is the last thing on athletes and parents mind when it comes to athletic performance and injury reduction. It seems that nutrition is often the missing piece to the performance and injury-reduction puzzle. Many young athletes mistakenly think that chugging an energy drink in the locker room before their match will help their performance. Or eating nothing for breakfast, then eating fast food for lunch, and then going to a two hour practice fueled by junk. Not really effective.

Think about this for a second, if young athletes are fueling themselves with junk and too little calories throughout the day, what effect do you think this will have on their performance on the field? Supportive nutrition fuels optimal performance and reduces injury potential in their sport by repairing muscles and improving health. If an athlete is not fueling properly with lean proteins, complex, good fats and adequately hydrating themselves with fluid, they will fatigue sooner in sport. They will never reach their true potential with their ACL reduction program. They will not optimally recover from practice to practice and after their games. This all will have a direct negative impact on their performance and chance of injury.

So there you have it, all six of these strategies must be implemented together. This is a recipe for success! If one ingredient is missing, then you reduce the effectiveness of the program while increasing the chance of injury of the young female athlete. Each strategy plays a vital role and are parts of a whole that when implemented together, will go a long way in preventing the high number of ACL injuries among the female high school athlete population.

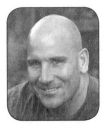

About Tim

Tim Rudd is the Co-Owner of Fit-2-The Core in Concord, CA. In 2005, Tim joined the elite ranks of the International Youth Conditioning Association. He has worked over the last several years with the organization to further his education in youth conditioning, performance and nutrition. The organization is renowned for paving the way for trainers, coaches and parents to revolutionize the way we condition our young athletes.

Tim has certifications from International Youth Conditioning Association in Youth Conditioning, Speed/Agility, High School Strength and Conditioning and Nutrition. Tim also has certifications from International Sports Sciences Association, and National Academy of Sports Medicine. He attended DVC while playing football and Cal State Hayward to pursue his Bachelor's Degree in Kinesiology.

Tim writes a column in *Sports Stars Magazine*, which is a magazine that covers youth sports in the San Francisco Bay Area. Tim covers training strategies for high school athletes. He is also a speaker and has presented his methodologies and best practices at numerous high schools throughout the Bay Area on the subject of injury prevention and athletic performance.

Tim currently works with young athletes from the ages of 12-18. His athletes include basketball, soccer, lacrosse, baseball, wrestling, MMA, football and volleyball players.

To learn more about Tim and his training programs go to: www.fasteryoungathletes.com for free videos on an array of subjects concerning youth performance.

CHAPTER 20

10 Steps To Improving Speed, Agility, And Coordination

By Corinne Briers

My heart is pounding. Thoughts are racing frantically through my head. I'm agonizing over every single play. Sitting there outside my coach's office patiently and nervously waiting for my turn, I'm a wreck! Most athletes dread sitting in their individual post-season meeting, facing their coach across that huge, intimidating desk. And I was no different. Playing soccer at my dream school, at one of the top programs in the country, and having just won the Pac-10 Championship, I was still incredibly anxious to hear what my coach had to say about the season.

"Well, Corinne...you're just not fast enough."

Without hesitation I replied, "Then I will become faster!"

But he insisted, "You can only become so fast, Corinne. You just weren't born with those genes."

Hmmmm....

Is it true? Am I never going to be an impact player at this level because I wasn't born fast?

So many coaches, parents, and athletes believe just that. Speed can't be taught. You are either born with it, or you are not. And it wasn't until I decided to go overseas and play professionally that I focused on truly developing my speed and realized that speed CAN be taught. Sure, there are always going to be players that are naturally gifted and ridiculously fast. But with the right technique and training, anyone can tap into his or her speed potential.

Luckily, I had a good friend that was rapidly becoming one of the best soccer performance specialists in the world and he trained me extensively. For the first time, I learned the technique of how to move efficiently, drive into the ground, change direction effectively, and get to the ball fast. It was amazing! Now, don't get me wrong, I didn't become 'wicked fast' all of a sudden. In fact, no one would ever use "fast" in describing me as a player. But what did happen was that speed was no longer an issue. In my pro career, "lack of speed" wasn't a weakness. Granted, I had other things I needed to improve, but I could definitely play at this level without every coach saying, "Corinne, you're just not fast enough."

It's kind of like singing. My mom has this incredible voice and my niece is extremely talented as well. Apparently the singing gene skipped a generation, however. If I try singing, windows crack. Seriously! If I went to a voice coach, however, and learned how to breathe properly and use my voice competently, I may not be recording albums any time soon, but I wouldn't need to mouth the words to Happy Birthday while everyone else is singing!

The moral of the story is that **speed can be taught.**

The Central Nervous System is constantly creating new pathways during youth developmental stages, so the younger you start developing speed, the better.

So, what can you do with your young athlete or team to improve speed?

Here are the 10 Steps to Improving Speed, Agility, and Coordination: a blueprint of specific activities and games you can implement immediately with your young athlete.

The best way to use this plan of action guide is to try it for 12 weeks. Perform the assessment on week 1 and again after week 12. Although it is difficult to determine which part of a young athlete's improvement is a result of specific training and which part is simply a result of growth and maturity, it is still important to get a baseline to know exactly where you are starting and how you improved.

In between the assessments, pick 1-2 exercises from the remaining 8 steps (steps 2-9) and perform them with your athlete about once a week. Training time should be between 30 minutes to 1 hour. Most importantly, make it fun! The more fun and enjoyable it is, the more the athlete will want to do it. I incorporated a bunch of game-like activities because kids of all ages enjoy those the most. They are not "little adults" that need to be trained like pro-athletes. Tap into the athlete's creativity and make it as fun and exciting as possible.

Please note that I have created a special webpage with pictures, videos, and explanations of these activities for readers of this book that need additional assistance or would like more detailed information on the *10 Steps To Improving Speed, Agility, and Coordination.* Go to www.AthleteDevelopmentAcademy.com/10steps.

STEP 1: ASSESSMENT

You can't know where you are going if you don't know where you are.

There are tons of assessment tests to choose from, so the criteria I used in selecting this list is based on little to no equipment, no specialized training necessary, and is easy to implement at a park or in a backyard or driveway.

Broad Jump – Standing 2-footed jump for distance. Measure from the start line to heel of closest foot to the line. Whichever body part is closest to the line gets measured, just like in the long jump. So try not to take a step back or fall backwards and put your hand down. Record best of 3 attempts.

20-yard sprint – Standing start. Timer starts on athlete's movement and stops when athlete hits the end line. Can be adapted to 40-yard sprint if testing an older athlete or if it is sport-related (i.e., baseball, track, etc). Record best of 3 attempts.

Obstacle Course/Relay Race – Allow a practice round to ensure athlete is familiar with the course. Time and record best of 2 attempts. (see Diagram 1)

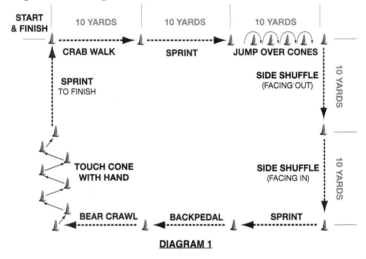

DIAGRAM 1

5-10-5 - A common agility shuttle test. Clock starts on athlete's first movement. Begin by straddling the line at middle cone (cone #1). Sprint from cone 1 to cone 2, touch the line, sprint from cone 2 to cone 3, touch the line, and then sprint through the finish at cone 1. Record two attempts. (Diagram 2)

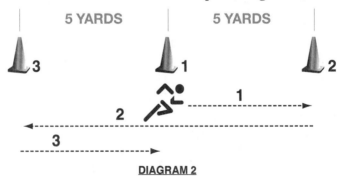

DIAGRAM 2

These tests can be applied to all ages. Choosing just the obstacle course would be sufficient for younger athletes.

An easy way to also make these tests qualitative is to simply film your athlete performing the assessment. Filming is an excellent way to see improvements in form and movement ability that timed scores fail to recognize. You don't need to be Steven Spielberg, just use your cell phone or video camera to capture how your athlete is moving. It doesn't take a highly-trained specialist to notice that an athlete is more coordinated, moving more efficiently, and looks more athletic while running.

STEP 2: BALANCE

Balance is a vital component to athletic development success. The objective is to improve body control and stability. This is especially important in young athletes due to their central nervous system constantly creating new neural pathways in the motor-control areas of the brain.

Here's Looking At You – Stand on one leg facing a partner, pick one person to lead and the other to follow. The person leading moves his or her hands and free leg in different directions anywhere they want, but SLOWLY. The follower is "mirroring" just like they are looking into a mirror and trying to stay balanced. Partners rotate roles and switch legs.

Balance Wars – Stand facing partner in a good athletic position with both hands raised in front of you at about shoulder height and palms facing partner. Object is to knock your partner off balance by either pushing against their hands or bringing your hands back towards you so they can't be pushed. You get a point for every time your partner loses balance and takes a step. First player to 5 points wins. Progress to one-legged balance wars.

Reverse Giant Walks – A backwards-walking lunge. Be sure to remind athlete to keep both feet facing forward and make sure front knee does not go past the toe of the front leg.

Hot Ballin' – 2 players, each standing on one leg, throw a ball back and forth. Challenge each other by throwing the ball high, low, hard, to the side, etc. Try to keep foot that is off the ground right next to the other foot but not touching it. So if needed, you can tap foot to the ground briefly to regain balance.

STEP 3: COORDINATION

The Central Nervous System (CNS) is in a state of constant development during the formative years of growth. There are sensitive periods within this CNS development that suggest it is imperative that youngsters be introduced to all sorts of stimuli to fuel improvements in coordination. Thus it is important to foster overall body awareness, synchronization of movement, and spatial awareness in developing athletes.

Jump Rope – One of the best tools to help develop body control and coordination in young athletes is the jump rope. The variations are endless. There are a ton of jump rope videos on YouTube if you are looking for ideas. And jumprope.com is a great resource too.

Follow-the-Leader – One player is the leader and one is the follower. The leader should do whatever they want and the follower needs to copy it. They can run, skip, turn in circles, somersault, cartwheel, do jumping jacks, etc. Encourage athletes to be silly and creative. Switch roles.

Skip To My Lou – Skipping variations include forward skips, backward skips, sideways skips with coordinated arm movement, forward or backward skips with opposite arm circles, high knee skips, low skips – just to name a few. Try them all!

Ladder, Ladder, Make It Matter – Ladder drills are a unique and fun way to develop coordination and sprint technique. My favorites are Ali-shuffle, icky-shuffle, reverse icky-shuffle, 2 feet in (linear and lateral), and 3-forward/1 back. Athlete should first attempt drills with arms on hips to learn the lower body footwork. When proficient, add the extra challenge of coordinating the arm movement.

STEP 4: MOBILITY & FLEXIBILITY

Mobility exercises dynamically stimulate the nervous system, muscles, tendons, and joints and prepare the body for the demands of sport. For youth athletes, these exercises also challenge balance, mobility, strength, coordination, and flexibility.

Crab Walk – Sit with feet on the ground facing forward and hands on the ground behind you (fingers facing forward), raise butt off the ground and walk forward using hands and feet. It's important to make sure athlete's feet are facing forward so the hamstrings can get activated.

Bear Crawl - Great for overall systemic strength and contrilateral coordination. Using only your hands and feet, crawl forward (or backwards) without allowing knees to touch the ground. These can be combined with the crab walk for a fun relay race too! Be creative!

Inch Worm – Start in a pushup position on the ground and while keeping your legs straight, walk your feet in towards your hands until you feel a good stretch on your hamstring. Then, walk your hands forward into a pushup position again. Repeat 5-10 times.

Puppy Crawls – In a crawling position on all fours, crawl forward a few steps and lift right leg up to the side (like a puppy peeing on a tree), bring it back to the middle and then lift leg behind you by pushing the heel up to the sky. Crawl forward a few more steps and repeat with the left leg. Repeat for 10-15 yards. An excellent activity for hip mobility and core stabilization.

STEP 5: STRENGTH

The stronger you are, the more force you can apply to the ground. The more force you can apply, the faster you will move. Therefore the training emphasis for most young athletes should be overall systemic strength and movement efficiency.

Leap Frog, Piggy Back & Wheel Barrel – Great systemic strength exercises that are super fun, and really challenging. Combine these classic childhood activities into a relay race that is sure to be a crowd favorite!

Monkey Bars – You'd be surprised to discover how many young athletes can't actually complete the monkey bars. This is a fun activity that is very useful in developing upper body strength. For older kids incorporate 30-second monkey bar holds (with straight extended arms – just hang), or monkey bar pull-up holds (where you hold at the top of the pull-up), and pull-ups or assisted pull-ups too.

Lava Rescue – Athlete jumps on your back and attempts to crawl all the way around you without touching the ground (or "lava") until he or she is back in the piggyback position again. Try again crawling around the other direction.

Slot Machine – Similar to Balance Wars in step 3, however partners clasp hands (like in arm wrestling) and push or pull to knock the other player off balance and force them to take a step. Use both right hands and left hands and progress to attempting it on only one leg.

Ballin' – Place a basket or trashcan in the middle of two participants 10-20 yards apart. Set up several balls (about 8-12 balls of different weights and sizes if possible) next to each athlete. Athletes must balance and stand on only one leg while reaching down to pick up one ball and try to throw it in the basket. Each successful throw into the basket equals one point. Competition ends when both athletes have thrown all of their balls. Athlete with the most points wins. Switch legs and play again.

Hot Hands – Both participants get in a pushup position facing each other. Attempt to tap/tag your partner's hands while avoiding getting yours tagged. One point for each successful tag. First player to 10 or 20 points wins. If too challenging, modify the pushup by placing knees on the ground.

STEP 6: TECHNIQUE

It's important to realize that with younger ages you simply want the athletes to explore the movement and not over-emphasize the technique. Introduce concepts during outcome-based activities that will allow the athlete to focus on the technique while playing. With older athletes you can concentrate more on the form and how they are moving. Try to connect an easily relatable concept to the actual movement you want the athlete to work on.

Gas Pedal – In sprinting, the arms are the gas pedal. The faster the arms move, the faster the legs move. Stand or sit and simply move the arms in a running motion. Go slow at first and then try to be as fast as possible. The arms remain slightly bent and hands should go in full range of motion between the eye socket and the hip pocket ("Hip to Lip" or "Cheek to cheek" are other common phrases used by track coaches). ...And try to keep the shoulders relaxed!

Freedom Runs – Stand with a wide stance behind the athlete and hold onto the front of his or her hips. Athlete sprints to cone 10 yards away while holder slowly walks forward (providing medium resistance to the sprinter). With the resistance, athlete must drive into the ground to propel forward. Remind athlete to keep ankle flexed, and push the ground away with the ball of the foot. Also, the higher they lift their leg, the harder they will be able to push into the ground and the more force they will generate to move faster. This can also occasionally progress to holding for 5 yards and then releasing the athlete to sprint on their own for 5-10 yards. Objective with the progression is to keep it fresh and fun, not actually conduct over-speed training.

STEP 7: SPEED

Speed is the ability to reach and maintain an optimum rate of motion. Better acceleration allows athletes to quickly get into positions to make plays. For younger kids try turning everyday activities or chores into fun speed activities. For example, time your athlete while taking out the trash, cleaning up his or her room, or running down the hall to put away clean laundry. Challenge them to beat their time.

Fetch N Furious – Two athletes lay down on stomach next to each other. From behind, throw two tennis balls in front of them at the same time. As soon as they see the ball, they should react immediately and sprint to get to it first. Can alter the starting position to sitting down with legs straight out in front, or lying on their backs.

Free Fallin' – Standing 5 yards away from partner, drop a tennis ball from shoulder height with an outstretched arm. As soon as ball is released, partner tries to sprint and grab it before it hits the ground a second time. Use various starting positions and different distances to challenge the athlete.

Rock, Paper, Scissor Sprints – Two athletes standing at cones 20 yards apart. They meet at the middle cone and perform rock, paper, scissors. The loser must turn and sprint back to his or her cone before getting tagged by the other athlete (winner). One point for every successful tag. First player to 5 points wins.

Mirror, Mirror – Two cones 15-20 yards apart. The line between the cones acts like a mirror. Partners face each other on either side of the line. One person is it and the other is the follower, mirroring the movement. The leader shuffles back and forth until deciding when to sprint to one of the two cones. The person mirroring needs to react quickly and try to be first to touch the cone instead. Switch roles.

STEP 8: AGILITY

Agility is the ability to move and change the direction and position of the body quickly and effectively while under control. The skills required to execute these movements depend on the development of several bio-motor abilities.

Agility has a more direct impact on sports performance than just pure speed. In fact, multi-directional movement ability is an essential element of athletic success. Improved performance depends largely on the athlete's ability to read the situation, make decisions, and react quickly.

Agility Tag – Partners attempt to tag each other's knee while avoiding getting their own knee tagged. Successful tag equals one point. Reset to a good athletic position after each score. First player to 5 points wins. Try Toe Tag too – where you attempt to tap your partner's foot with yours while avoiding getting your own toes tagged.

The Get Away – One person is the chaser, and other person is getting away. On "go" a player tries to get away from the chaser by running all over and changing direction quickly. The chaser tries to stay as close to the player as possible. On "freeze" the athletes stop moving immediately. If the chaser can touch the athlete getting away, it equals 1 point (allow younger athletes to take a giant leap before trying to touch partner to get a point). Switch roles.

The Great Escape – make an obstacle course that incorporates several components of speed, agility, and coordination. Have the athlete help create it. Or use the diagram from the assessment to generate ideas. (Diagram 1)

I Got Your Back – Two athletes 30 yards apart. Mark each starting line with cones placed 10 yards apart. Player A is the attacker and player B is the tagger. Player A attempts to run past player B and across the opposite line without getting his or her back tagged. If successful, player A gets a point. No point awarded if player A runs out of bounds or if player B tags the athlete's back. Switch roles. First player to 10 points wins.

STEP 9: PLAY ANOTHER SPORT

Playing another sport is an excellent way to help the developing athlete efficiently improve overall athletic skill. Brian Grasso, founder of the International Youth Conditioning Association, shared a great analogy explaining the importance of playing multiple sports and avoiding overtraining. He explained that if your child is really good at math, you wouldn't forget all about History, English, and Science class and instead sign up for math camp and everything you can find that's math-related. You wouldn't dream of doing this because you understand that your child's brain needs English, reading, science, and history to fully develop. Yet when a child is great at one sport we forget about everything else and sign up for only soccer- related activities (or football, or baseball, etc.). So please encourage your athlete to play multiple sports throughout the year.

STEP 10: POST ASSESSMENT

Repeat the initial assessment from step 1. Recognize that athletic development is a long-term process. From the assessment find positives so the kids may focus on the success and feel more confident about the work they've put in.

Remember, if you need additional assistance, go to: www.AthleteDevelopmentAcademy.com/10steps

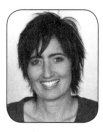

About Corinne

Corinne Briers has played professionally on some of the top women's soccer teams in the world and was a starter for her National Team. She even played professionally in Sweden for Pia Sundhage, who is the current coach of the U.S. Women's National Team. Corinne grew up playing in Southern California and went on to play for USC where she won the PAC-10 Championship. Corinne has high level coaching licenses from 3 different countries and was on the coaching staff for one of only 7 teams in the Women's Professional Soccer League in the U.S.

Corinne has worked with youth of all ages for over 12 years and is the founder and director of the Athlete Development Academy. Her coaching and unique understanding of kids and teens allows athletes to tap into their potential both on and off the field.

Through the world-renowned International Youth Conditioning Association, Corinne is a Certified Youth Fitness Specialist, Youth Speed and Agility Specialist, High School Strength and Conditioning Coach, and Youth Nutrition Specialist.

In addition to her expertise in helping mold young athletes and soccer players into better athletes, Corinne is also a Certified Life Coach and Goal Setting expert. She is the founder of Teen Results, a place where her passion helps teens develop habits to make a lasting impression on their lives. And Corinne is a sought-after keynote speaker, where she shares her inspiring story to aid the audience in learning tools and strategies to deal with life's challenges.

To learn more about Corinne Briers visit
www.AthleteDevelopmentAcademy.com
and www.CorinneBriers.com.

CHAPTER 21

5 Steps to Reducing Non-Contact ACL Injuries in Female Athletes

By David Kittner

LINDSAY'S TRAGEDY

She had all the makings of having an outstanding college softball career and was in a position to write her own ticket to the school of her choice – until that fateful day in the high school gymnasium. Lindsay Roy, of Brampton, Ontario, was a prominent softball pitcher from the first day she began playing organized sports at the age of six. An exceptional athlete, Lindsay played numerous sports as a child though softball was her true love. Lindsay rose through the ranks of her local girls' softball league establishing her as a premier pitcher.

As a senior in high school, Lindsay attracted lots of attention from colleges and universities from across North America. Schools were knocking on her door with offerings of scholarship monies beyond her wildest dreams. However in March 2001, at only 18 years of age, any thoughts of playing college softball came to a crashing halt. In her high school's gymnasium Lindsay was performing running long jump for her high school's track and field team. On one of her jumps, Lindsay landed awkwardly and immediately felt a sharp pain in her left knee.

The pain was unlike anything Lindsay had ever experienced before. She knew from the awkwardness of her landing and from the intense pain she was feeling, something was seriously wrong. Although Lindsay was able to get up and walk, albeit gingerly, things would spiral downward for her from that point forward. In the days that followed, Lindsay's knee had swollen to unprecedented proportions.

After numerous trips to over ten different medical professionals Lindsay was diagnosed with a torn anterior cruciate ligament, (ACL). Lindsay endured reparative surgery, and months and months of intensive rehabilitation that was emotionally, mentally and physically draining on both her and her family. As if this wasn't difficult enough, Lindsay found herself facing another dilemma; the schools that had been wooing her for the past two years suddenly stopped calling and lost interest.

In the years that followed, Lindsay required additional surgeries and continued intensive rehabilitation. Along the way, she tore the ACL in her right knee. Now, as an adult, with her competitive youth athletic career long over, Lindsay continues to battle issues resulting from her ACL injuries. Though she remains hopeful that someday she will be able to compete again as an adult, the effect of the injuries are currently felt daily as Lindsay works to recover.

It's not a stretch to say that the day Lindsay tore her ACL was a life-changing event. Aside from her current struggle to rehabilitate both knees, simple daily activities remain a challenge. In addition, Lindsay is now at risk for degenerative knee issues in the future.

Lindsay's story is not unique. Young female athletes just like Lindsay continue to suffer non-contact ACL injuries on a daily basis. Sadly, many of these injuries can be avoided. Let's take a closer look as to why stories like Lindsay's are so common.

WHAT IT IS, WHAT IT DOES,
AND HOW IT'S INJURED

The Anterior Cruciate Ligament (ACL) is one of four main ligaments in the knee joint that collectively with the Medial Collateral Ligament (MCL), the Lateral Collateral Ligament (LCL) and the Posterior Cruciate Ligament, connects the lower leg (shin bones - tibia and fibula) to the upper leg (thigh bone - femur). The ACL and PCL cross each other inside the knee, forming an "X." This is why they're called the "Cruciate" (cross-like) ligaments. The role of these four ligaments is to provide stability to the knee during movement.

There are two types of ACL injuries; contact and non-contact. A blow to the side of the knee resulting from a tackle or fall is an example of a contact ACL injury. Non-contact ACL injuries occur when an athlete comes to a quick stop combined with a change of direction on one leg or is landing from a jump as was the case with Lindsay. This is why soccer, lacrosse, field hockey, volleyball and basketball have the highest incidences of non-contact ACL injuries.

Female teenage athletes between the ages of 13 and 18 are four to eight times more susceptible to injuring their ACLs than their male teenage counterparts. The higher incidence of non-contact ACL injuries in girls than boys can be attributed to things going on outside the body as well as inside the body. External factors include the interactions between the athlete's shoes and the surface upon which they are playing, the type of surface being played on, and the weather. Internal factors include anatomical, neuromuscular, biomechanical, and hormonal factors.

SO WHAT CAN BE DONE?

Since many of the aforementioned factors cannot be changed, it only makes sense to focus on those factors that can be changed and improved upon: the biomechanical and neuromuscular systems.

Let's look at the biomechanical specifics:

1. Females have wider hips than boys thus creating a sharper angle, known as the Q angle. This is measurement of the angle between the Quadriceps (Rectus Femoris is usually used) and the patella tendon. The greater the angle, the greater the pressure applied to the inside of their knees.

2. Females have a greater quadricep to hamstring ratio causing a muscle imbalance as their quadriceps overpower their hamstrings during movements. The imbalances created by the overpowering quadriceps creates added stress on the ACL.

3. Females tend to play sports in a more upright position and land or cut and change direction with stiffer legs, thereby reducing the amount of hamstring and glute activation needed to protect the knee.

4. Females have a narrower intercondylar notch. The intercondylar notch is a small groove in the femur whereby the ACL travels. Because the intercondylar notch is smaller, the ACL is more susceptible to being stressed as the knee moves, especially during twisting or hyperextension movements.

5. The ligaments of females have more give than men's. Also, women's muscle tissue is more elastic than males. Combine excessive joint motion with increased flexibility and you have greater stress on the ACL.

Contributing factors such as gender, Q angles, intercondylar notch size, and ligament laxity cannot be changed or controlled. However, what can be controlled is the level of quality training your athletes receive on a year-round basis.

While there is no singular program or training protocol that can prevent all non-contact ACL injuries, much can be done from a training perspective to reduce the possibilities of one happening.

Training programs that incorporate exercises that mimic sport, instead of relying on isolative exercises, (we've all seen athletes sitting at a machine and working one muscle at a time) are imperative. Think about training the kinetic chain with an emphasis on the ankles, knees, hips, and core. In addition, it is extremely important for female athletes to learn how to execute movement patterns such as jumping, landing, stopping and changing direction. An athlete may be fit, but if they have not established safe movement patterns, they remain highly susceptible to non-contact ACL injuries.

For the female athlete, training year round is not an option, it's a necessity. A recent report released by the National Strength and Conditioning Association reveals that implementing an effective year-round training program has been shown to minimize peak landing forces by 22% and reduce ACL injuries by 88% in younger athletes. Effective training means using a systemic, progressive approach.

FIVE EASY STEPS

STEP #1: Warm-up

The purpose of the warm-up is to prepare the athlete for the work to follow whether it is a workout, practice or game. Every workout, practice and game should be preceded by a thorough warm-up to prepare the athletes for the work to follow and to help reduce incidences of ACL injuries. Warming up improves tissue quality, dynamic flexibility, proprioception, increases the body's core temperature, increases blood flow and increases breathing rate throughout the body. A proper warm-up would include but not be limited to the following:

A. Tissue Quality and Mobility
- Foam rolling
- Ankle mobility
- Hip mobility
- Thoracic spine mobility
- One legged balancing

B. General Warm-up
- Forward run
- Backward run
- Forward skipping
- Backward skipping
- Carioca
- Side Shuffle

C. Dynamic Warm-up
- Knee hugs
- Heel to butt
- Straight leg kicks
- Leg cradles
- Forward lunges
- Rear Lunges

Step #2: Stability and Eccentric Strength

Developing stability and eccentric strength (the ability to land and absorb force) follows the warm-up. Learning to land correctly from a two foot jump and a one foot hop in multiple directions is an important skill in developing ACL injury resistance in young female athletes. Make sure that you start slow and low. For maximum benefit and to prevent injuries in training, it is extremely important to be progressive with the chosen exercises and not over do it. Technique in each of the exercises and movements is essential.

Jumps (two feet, saggital and frontal planes)
- Two foot jump up onto a box with a step down
- Two foot jump over a hurdle. Start low, 3-6 inches
- Two foot jump over hurdles with a bounce
- Two foot jump over hurdles but remove bounce and add

in elasticity

Hops (one foot, saggital and frontal planes)
- One foot hop onto a box with a step down
- One foot hop over a hurdle
- One foot hop over hurdles with a bounce
- One foot hop over hurdles but remove bounce and add in elasticity

Step #3: Strength

The key to effective strength development is to use a non-machine, single leg, progressive approach including both knee and hip dominant exercises. Like all exercises, progression and technique is important. Below are three examples of single leg knee-dominant and single leg hip-dominant exercises:

Single Leg Knee-Dominant Exercises
- Lunges
- Squats
- Box Step Ups

Single Leg Hip-Dominant Exercises
- Hip Bridges
- Deadlifts
- Good mornings

Step #4: Change of Direction

The concept of changing directions is a critical component of the training paradigm. The goal is for your athletes to establish effective and correct movement patterns so those same movement patterns can be repeated automatically on the field or court. Skills involving deceleration, such as forward lunge stops, reverse lunge stops, angled stops, split stops and shuttle stops are all key components to developing correct and safe movement patterns.

Deceleration movement skills are taught in a progressive manner beginning with static repeats then moving on to dynamic repeats, random repeats, predictable specificity repeats and random specificity repeats.

Step #5: Energy Systems Conditioning

Energy systems conditioning plays a huge role in training and development. Linear conditioning may be appropriate for athletes who participate in linear-type sports like track and field, but there aren't many sports where linear conditioning alone will be of much use. When preparing your athletes for multi-directional sports, it only makes sense your conditioning programs include multi-directional movement with stops and starts. Some examples of lateral conditioning include shuttle runs, skater hops and slide boards.

A DIFFERENT ENDING?

While non-contact ACL injuries cannot be prevented, much can be accomplished away from the playing fields to minimize the risk in your athletes. When programming effective training with progressive skill development, your athletes will become injury resistant and better performers on and off the field.

The time and effort invested in a year-round training and development program for young female athletes far outweighs the emotional, mental and physical trauma they will encounter when a non-contact ACL injury occurs. Lindsay's injury not only halted a promising collegiate athletic career, but continues to affect her emotionally, mentally and physically on a daily basis. There is no "magic bullet" training program that will prevent non-contact ACL injuries. There are, however, research-driven protocols as outlined above, that coaches responsible for training young female athletes need to follow in order to reduce the number of non-contact ACL injuries in female athletes. These protocols represent what is known in the strength and conditioning field as good training.

As a coach, seek out individuals certified as youth training and fitness specialists to work with your athletes on an annual basis. It could very well be the difference in the type of story your athletes tells versus the story Lindsay tells.

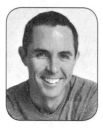

About David

David Kittner, aka the Youth Fitness Guy, is a passionate, caring and dedicated individual with over 20 years experience working with children. He truly understands the unique sciences associated with child development and the practical means by which those must be applied to any fitness or sport-based venture.

He is among the leading authorities of more than 2,500 Youth Fitness Specialists that make up the International Youth Conditioning Association, the premier international authority with respect to athletic development and youth-participant-based conditioning.

David is certified as a Youth Fitness Specialist, Youth Speed and Agility Specialist, and a Youth Nutrition Specialist with the International Youth Conditioning Association.

David conducts athletic development sessions, workshops and clinics for youth athletes, parents, teachers and coaches, and presents at Fitness and Physical Education conferences. He also serves as Education Director for SchoolFit, Youth Fitness Specialist and Master Trainer for Lebert Fitness and Youth Strength and Conditioning Coach for the Fitness nation.

David resides in Brampton, Ontario with his two active children, Julia and Thomas.

To request an interview or to get in touch with David, please contact him by phone at: 647-504-7638 or by e-mail at: david@youthfitnessguy.com